Laparoscopic Surgery of the Spleen

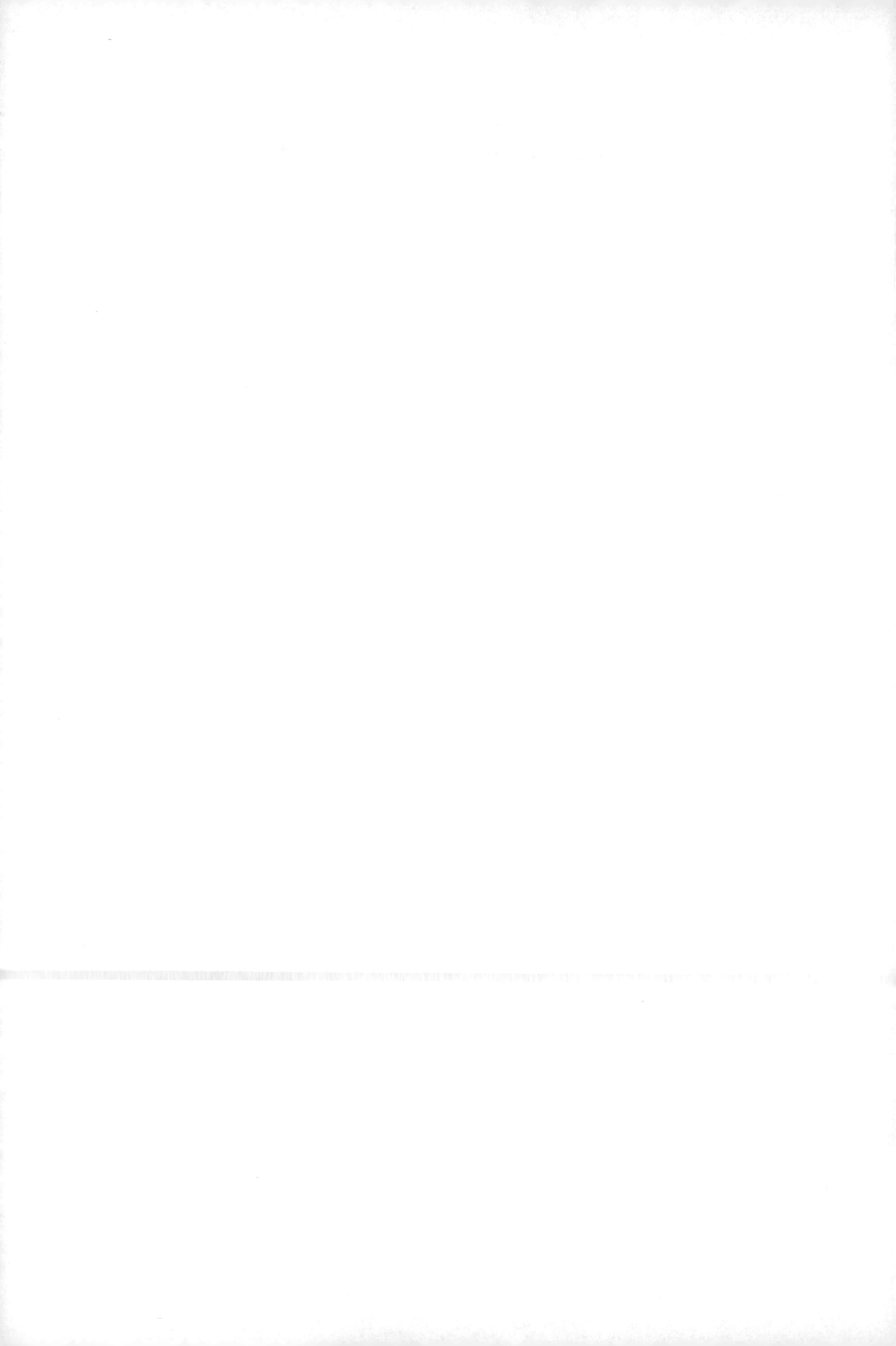

Bing Peng
Editor

Laparoscopic Surgery of the Spleen

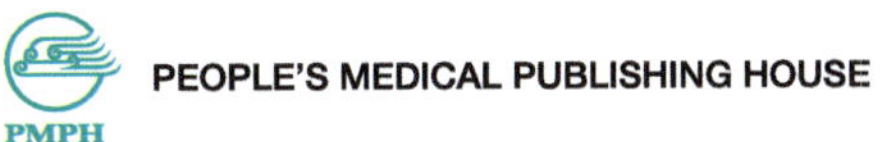

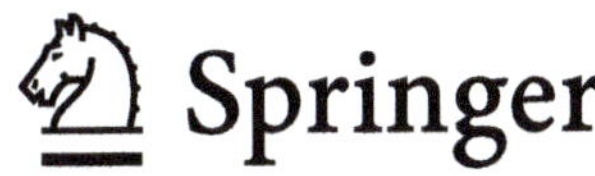

Editor
Bing Peng
HPB Minimally Invasive Surgery
West China Hospital of Sichuan University
Chengdu
Sichuan
China

ISBN 978-981-16-1218-3 ISBN 978-981-16-1216-9 (eBook)
https://doi.org/10.1007/978-981-16-1216-9
Jointly published with People's Medical Publishing House, PR of China.

This Springer imprint is published by the registered company Springer Nature Singapore Pte Ltd.
The registered company address is: 152 Beach Road, #21-01/04 Gateway East, Singapore 189721, Singapore

Foreword

This book summarizes the clinical experience and scientific research achievements of the author's team, with reference to the latest important literatures and monographs published at home and abroad, and illustrates the key techniques, operation difficulties, and perioperative management for laparoscopic spleen surgery. I had the honor to read this book, which impressed me a lot. First of all, I would like to express my appreciation to the editor-in-chief and the author's excellent skills and advanced philosophy of minimally invasive surgery. Secondly, the pictures in this book are elaborate and vivid, fully reflecting their masterly skills in this field. Finally, it is worth noting that the invaluable experience shown in this book is exactly what readers are currently looking for. I believe that this book will provide theoretical support and technical guidance for young and middle-aged surgeons to carry out laparoscopic spleen surgery in a standardized manner.

Harbin, Heilongjiang, China
May 2018

Hongchi Jiang
First Affiliated Hospital of
Harbin Medical University
Harbin, China

Chinese Association of Surgeons
Beijing, China

Chinese Medical Doctor Association
Beijing, China

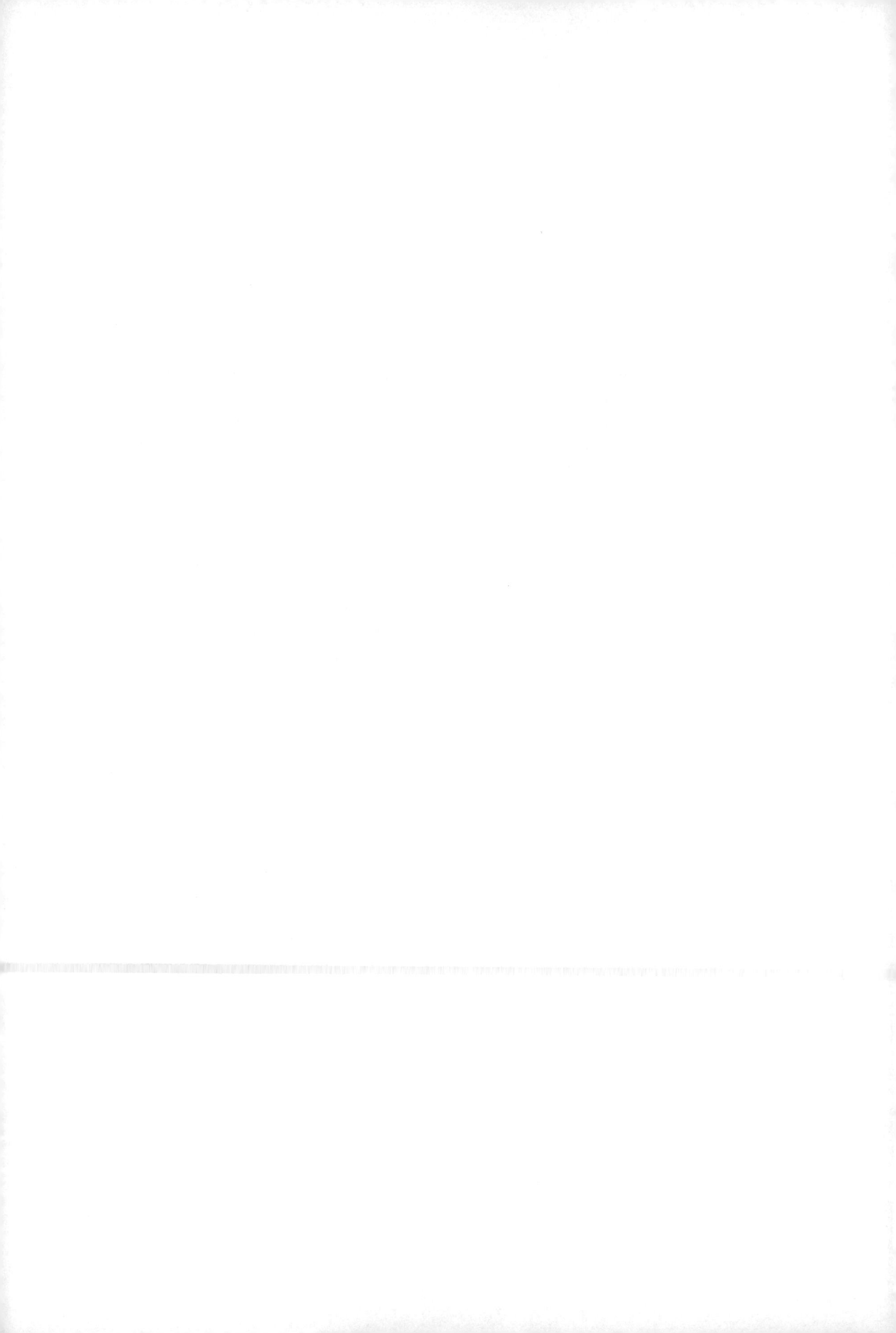

Preface

Spleen surgery is an old discipline that dates back to the sixteenth century in Europe. It came into existence in 1549 when the Italian surgeon Zaccarello successfully completed the first splenectomy. For more than 400 years since then, abdominal splenectomy has been the standard procedure for the treatment of spleen-related diseases.

Minimally invasive techniques have been extensively applied to each field of general surgery since the 1980s. An example is the laparoscopic technique, which has become the first choice in surgery due to its advantages such as less intraoperative bleeding, smaller wound, light postoperative pain at the wound, shorter hospital stay, and good cosmetic effect.

The technique has been accepted and recognized by most surgeons in consideration of its safety and feasibility since the first laparoscopic splenectomy case was reported in 1991 by Delaitre and Maignien in France. Spleen is considered as a parenchymatous organ most suitable for laparoscopic excision as no postoperative reconstruction is needed and the anatomical position of the spleen is fixed, just like appendectomy and gallbladder surgery.

Generally, the indications of laparoscopic splenectomy are the same as those of open splenectomy, except for the controversial splenic trauma. Currently, splenectomy is mainly carried out for spleen-related benign blood diseases, spleen-related malignant blood diseases, and space-occupying lesion of spleen.

As a key procedure of precise laparoscopic splenectomy, it is important to measure the volume of the spleen with abdominal ultrasound. High-resolution enhanced CT should be performed as a routine before splenectomy for blood diseases to detect the existence of the accessory spleen. The accessory spleen should be excised in order to achieve a good therapeutic effect. Foreign scholars also recommend vaccines against *S. pneumoniae*, *H. influenzae*, and *N. meningitidis* 15 days before the surgery to prevent postoperative infections.

Laparoscopic splenectomy can be carried out under supine position, semilateral position, and lateral decubitus position. These positions have their advantages and disadvantages, which are mainly determined by the surgeon's habits and clinical experience.

Hand-assisted laparoscopic splenectomy is particularly suitable for megalosplenia with a longitudinal diameter over 22 cm or a transverse diameter over 19 cm as it combines the techniques of open and laparoscopic splenectomy. The surgery allows easy bleeding control, ensures a relatively low conversion rate, shortens the operation duration and length of stay, alleviates postoperative pain, and is conducive to earlier food-taking.

Compared with traditional laparoscopic splenectomy, single-port laparoscopic splenectomy can achieve better minimally invasive results despite the equal intraoperative conversion rate, incidence of postoperative complications, and mortality. But with the improvement in technical devices and accumulation of surgeons' experience, the operation will definitely be promoted and popularized in the near future.

One of the essential principles of minimally invasive surgery is preservation of the organ. With the in-depth understanding of surgical anatomy and physiological functions of the spleen, laparoscopic partial splenectomy has become the first choice for treatment of space-occupying lesion. It also conforms to the concept of precise surgery.

Of course, we should be alert to the severe complications after splenectomy, such as postoperative thrombosis at the splenic vein or portal vein, especially at the portal vein, which may cause deterioration of liver function, gastrointestinal bleeding, intestinal ischemia, and even necrosis. In addition, routine postoperative anticoagulation should be performed for high-risk patients as thrombosis is related to the systemic coagulation condition and is positively correlated with splenic vein diameter and spleen size. Anticoagulation right after thrombosis can often achieve favorable vascular recanalization rate. Another complication is overwhelming post-splenectomy infection (OPSI), whose manifestations include systemic mucocutaneous hemorrhage and disseminated or diffuse intravascular coagulation (DIC) with no clear infection site. Preoperative vaccines mentioned above can significantly reduce the risk of OPSI. Laparoscopic splenectomy does not reduce the risk of the relative OPSI though it can significantly control postoperative infection at the wound.

Since the beginning of the twenty-first century, we have completed nearly 800 cases of laparoscopic spleen surgery and also accumulated some clinical experience. We have published more than 40 journal articles related to the spleen, among which about 30 were included in SCI. Besides, we have reported the first single-port laparoscopic splenectomy in China and first proposed the laparoscopic splenectomy using the superior approach, which makes the operation safe and feasible and reduces the conversion rate and the risk of complications. According to clinical practice and authoritative publications, we proposed that preoperative or intraoperative platelet transfusion is not necessary for patients with immune thrombocytopenic purpura and an extremely low blood platelet level, even lower than 1×10^9/L, if their coagulation functions are normal. Therefore, a blood platelet level even lower than 20×10^9/L is no longer the absolute contraindication of splenectomy as long as the coagulation function is normal, which has gained international recognition.

There are reasons to believe that laparoscopic splenectomy will become a standard procedure for the treatment of any diseases requiring splenectomy in the near future with the technical development and accumulation of surgeons' experience. Currently, there is no monograph in China systematically describing laparoscopic spleen surgery. Although most Grade-III Class-A hospitals can carry out laparoscopic spleen surgery, some surgeons in some hospitals may not be aware of the standard operation procedures. As such, we have compiled this book with reference to the relative literatures, focusing on the key points and difficulties (including perioperative management) of laparoscopic spleen surgery. We also included our own experience and pictures. After numerous times of modification in more than 1 year, we have completed this book with the diligence and intelligence of our team. Please be noted that there might be some mistakes and deficiencies in this book due to limitation of our experience, knowledge, and skills. Any criticism or correction is welcomed. We hope that by means of publication and dissemination of this book we can contribute to the development of laparoscopic spleen surgery in China, even a small step, toward standardization.

Chengdu, Sichuan, China
May 2018

Bing Peng

Contents

1 **Overview and Prospects of Laparoscopic Splenectomy** 1
Xiaodong Chen, Shi Qiu, and Bing Peng

2 **Anatomy and Physiology of the Spleen** 21
Guoqing Ouyang, Wanlong Wu, and Bing Peng

3 **Pathology and Pathophysiology of Surgical Spleen Diseases** ... 35
He Cai, Junhe Gou, Qijun Chen, and Bing Peng

4 **Perioperative Management of Laparoscopic Splenic Surgery and Application of Enhanced Recovery After Surgery (ERAS)** 51
Yunqiang Cai, Lingwei Meng, Man Zhang, and Bing Peng

5 **Laparoscopic Splenectomy (LS)** 59
Lingwei Meng, Sirui Chen, Bo Liao, Chunlin Li, and Bing Peng

6 **Single Incision Laparoscopic Splenectomy (SILS)** 73
Shuodong Wu, Runwen Liu, and Ying Fan

7 **Hand-Assisted Laparoscopic Splenectomy** 85
Hua Zhang, Yichao Wang, and Bing Peng

8 **Laparoscopic Partial Splenectomy** 93
Yongbin Li, Xin Wang, Junfeng Wang, Ke Chen, and Bing Peng

9 **Laparoscopic Splenectomy Combined Selective Pericardial Devascularization** 103
Yongbin Li, Xin Wang, Haojun Wu, Jun Xu, Jiaying You, and Bing Peng

10 **Laparoscopic Radical Antegrade Modular Pancreatosplenectomy** 113
Pan Gao, Aihua Dong, and Bing Peng

Correction to: Overview and Prospects of Laparoscopic Splenectomy C1
Xiaodong Chen, Shi Qiu, and Bing Peng

Index 125

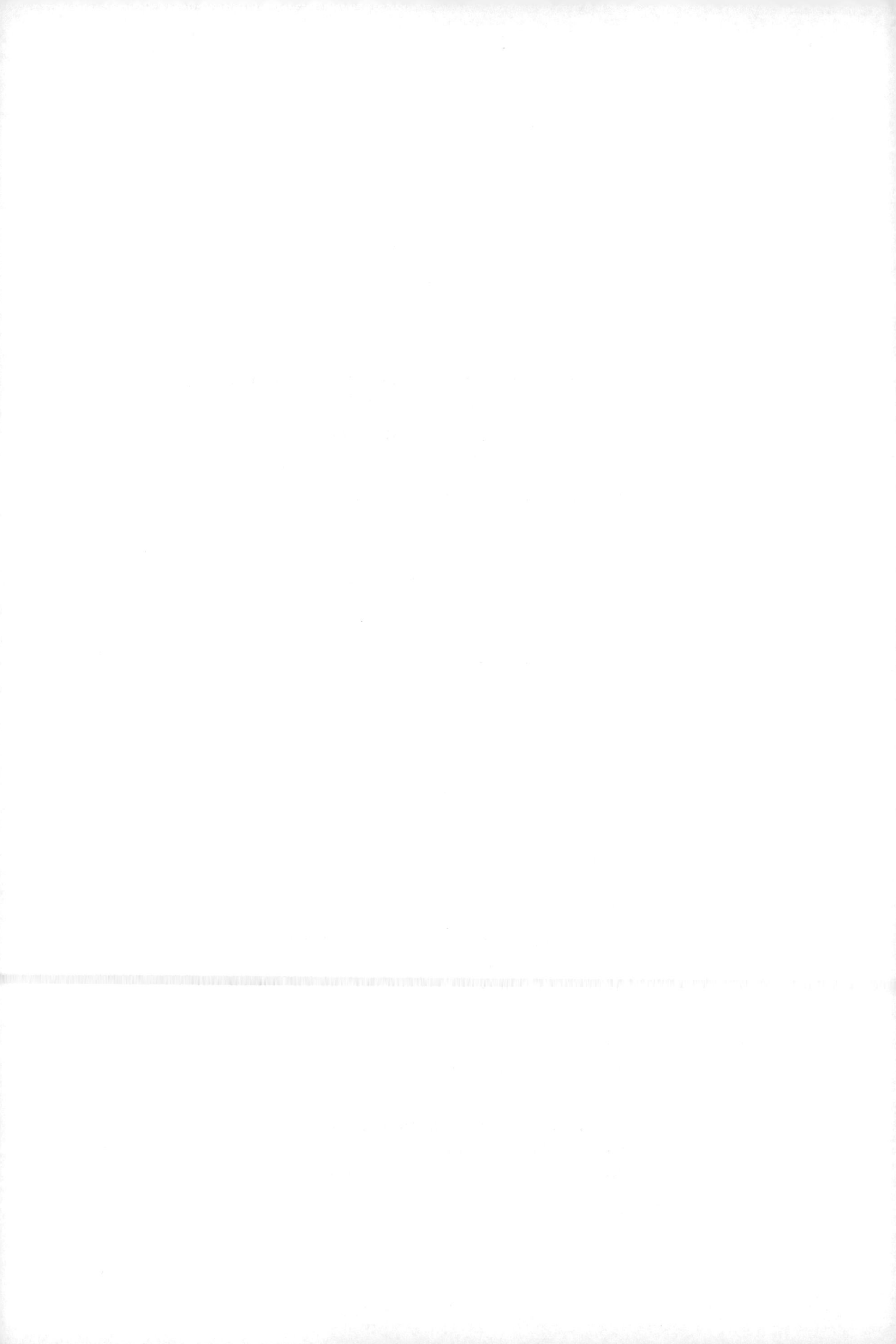

About the Editor

About the Editor

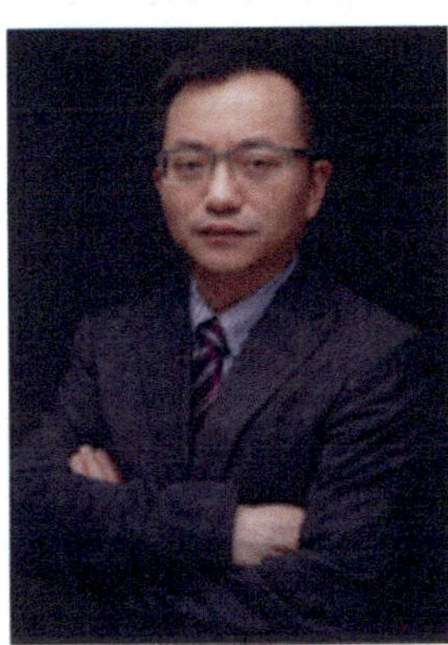

Bing Peng, M.D. works as a Chief Physician as well as a professor and a doctoral supervisor for the Pancreatic Surgery Department of West China Hospital, Sichuan University. He received his bachelor's degree of clinical medicine from the Medical College of Soochow University in July 1989 and doctor's degree of surgery from the West China Center of Medical Sciences, Sichuan University, in July 1996. Dr. Peng learned from Professor Wu Yantao and Professor Wu Heguang—renowned liver, gall, pancreas, and spleen surgical experts, and studied in the School of Medicine, Johann Wolfgang Goethe-Universität Frankfurt am Main. Now, he is a Fellow of the American College of Surgeons; Fellow of the International Association of Surgeons, Gastroenterologists and Oncologists (IASGO); Member of IASGO Minimally Invasive Surgery China Branch; Member of the Chinese Society of Laparoscopic and Endoscopic Surgery, Chinese Surgical Society, Chinese Medical Association; Member of Society of Minimally Invasive Surgery, Chinese College of Surgeons, Chinese Medical Doctor Association; Vice Director of Minimally Invasive Treatment for Pancreatic Cancer, Pancreatic Cancer Committee of Chinese Anti-Cancer Association; Vice Director of Minimally Invasive Treatment for Pancreatic Diseases, Society of Pancreatic Diseases, China International Exchange and Promotive Association for Medical and Health Care; Vice Chairman of Professional Committee of Abdominal Oncology, Chinese Medical Education Association; Member of Chinese

Endoscopic Doctors Association, Chinese Medical Doctor Association; and Director of the Preparatory Group of Professional Committee of Pancreatic Disease, Sichuan Medical Doctor Association.

Dr. Peng has been dedicated to the basic and clinical work in minimally invasive liver, biliary, pancreas, and spleen surgery, especially in spleen surgery. He is the first one to carry out and promote laparoscopic partial splenectomy, and the first one around the globe to propose that laparoscopic splenectomy is safe and feasible for patients with immune thrombocytopenic purpura and an extremely low blood platelet level if their coagulation functions are normal. In addition, he is the first one in China to carry out the highly difficult totally laparoscopic pancreatoduodenectomy, which initiated and promoted the second wave of the operation in China, and he takes the lead in China to carry out laparoscopic pancreatoduodenectomy combined with superior mesenteric (portal) vein resection, autologous blood vessel transplantation, and artificial blood vessel replacement. He has been invited many times to demonstrate laparoscopic pancreatoduodenectomy in China and abroad (Russia) and has been highly praised for that.

He has presided over or participated in 6 national and provincial scientific research projects, published more than 60 journal articles on domestic and overseas academic journals as the first author or corresponding author, among which nearly 30 articles on the spleen were included in SCI, and acted as the editor-in-chief of *Laparoscopic Spleen Surgery* (published by People's Health Publishing House).

In addition, he was also an editorial board member or reviewer for *Translational Cancer Research (TCR)*, *World Journal of Hepatology*, *World Journal of Gastroenterology*, *Chinese Journal of Laparoscopic Surgery*, *Chinese Journal of Bases and Clinics in General Surgery*, *Journal of Laparoscopic Surgery*, and *Journal of Hepatopancreatobiliary Surgery.*

Editors and Contributors

Associate Editors

Xiaodong Chen Sichuan Cancer Hospital, School of Medicine, University of Electronic Science and Technology of China, Chengdu, China

Yongbin Li West China Hospital, Sichuan University, Chengdu, China

Contributors

He Cai West China Hospital, Sichuan University, Chengdu, China

Yunqiang Cai West China Hospital, Sichuan University, Chengdu, China

Ke Chen West China Hospital, Sichuan University, Chengdu, China

Qijun Chen West China Second University Hospital, Sichuan University, Chengdu, China

Sirui Chen Mianyang Center Hospital, Mianyang, China

Xiaodong Chen Sichuan Cancer Hospital, School of Medicine, University of Electronic Science and Technology of China, Chengdu, China

Aihua Dong West China Hospital, Sichuan University, Chengdu, China

Ying Fan Shengjing Hospital of China Medical University, Shenyang, China

Pan Gao West China Hospital, Sichuan University, Chengdu, China

Junhe Gou West China Hospital, Sichuan University, Chengdu, China

Chunlin Li Cinical Medical College & Affiliated Hospital of Chengdu University, Chengdu, China

Yongbin Li West China Hospital, Sichuan University, Chengdu, China

Bo Liao AVIC 363 Hospital, Chengdu, China

Runwen Liu West China Hospital, Sichuan University, Chengdu, China

Lingwei Meng West China Hospital, Sichuan University, Chengdu, China

Guoqing Ouyang West China Hospital, Sichuan University, Chengdu, China

Bing Peng West China Hospital, Sichuan University, Chengdu, China

Shi Qiu West China Hospital, Sichuan University, Chengdu, China

Junfeng Wang The First People's Hospital of Yunnan Province, Kunming, China

Xin Wang West China Hospital, Sichuan University, Chengdu, China

Yichao Wang West China Hospital, Sichuan University, Chengdu, China

Haojun Wu West China Hospital, Sichuan University, Chengdu, China

Shuodong Wu Shengjing Hospital of China Medical University, Shenyang, China

Wanlong Wu West China Hospital, Sichuan University, Chengdu, China

Jun Xu West China Hospital, Sichuan University, Chengdu, China

Jiaying You West China Hospital, Sichuan University, Chengdu, China

Hua Zhang West China Hospital, Sichuan University, Chengdu, China

Man Zhang West China Hospital, Sichuan University, Chengdu, China

1 Overview and Prospects of Laparoscopic Splenectomy

Xiaodong Chen, Shi Qiu, and Bing Peng

1.1 Overview

Since it was first reported in 1991, laparoscopic splenectomy (LS) has been extensively performed in clinical practices worldwide. Over the past three decades, it has addressed more and more indications, covering almost all diseases in need of splenectomy by virtue of ever-improving surgical skills. Therefore, LS has been widely accepted as the "standard procedure" of splenectomy [1, 2].

When the keywords "laparoscopic splenectomy" were searched in PubMed, it was found that 1969 articles, including some not typical LS, had been released from January 1, 1991, to December 31, 2017. Nevertheless, only one article on laparoscopic splenectomy [3] was available in 1991, and the number of articles had been increasing steadily year by year ever since then (Fig. 1.1). Among these articles, Chinese scholars contributed 165, accounting for 8.4% of the total number, and we published 27 [4–30], accounting for 16.4% of the total number of Chinese articles.

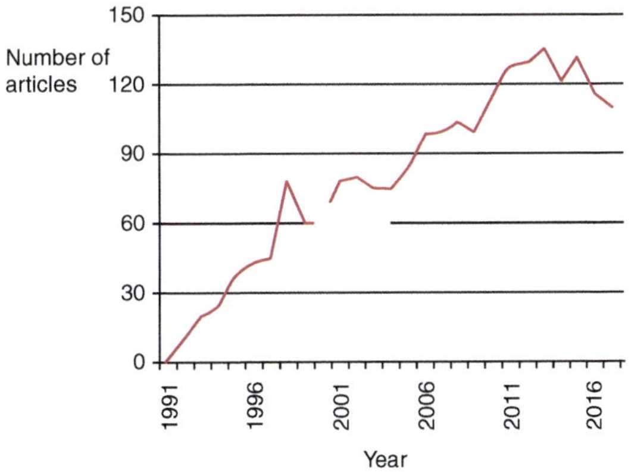

Fig. 1.1 Number of articles on LS in PubMed from 1991 to 2017

In this chapter, we will review the crucial findings in literatures of high-level evidence, including randomized controlled trials (RCT), meta-analysis (MA), systematic reviews (SR), and clinical practice guidelines (CPG). Meanwhile, we will also discuss the present situation, hot topics, and controversial issues and look into the future of laparoscopic splenectomy in combination with our own clinical experience and research results.

1.2 Indications

In general, the indications of LS are consistent with those of open splenectomy (OS). We started to promote LS in 2003, and a total of 302 cases

The original version of this chapter was revised. A correction to this chapter is available at https://doi.org/10.1007/978-981-16-1216-9_11

X. Chen
Sichuan Cancer Hospital, School of Medicine, University of Electronic Science and Technology of China, Chengdu, China

S. Qiu · B. Peng (✉)
West China Hospital, Sichuan University, Chengdu, China

B. Peng (ed.), *Laparoscopic Surgery of the Spleen*, https://doi.org/10.1007/978-981-16-1216-9_1

Table 1.1 Indications and main clinical characteristics of 302 patients receiving LS

Indications	Case No.	Sex (M/F)	Age (years)	ASA	Spleen size (cm)
Total	302	113/189	41 ± 16	2.1 ± 0.5	16.8 ± 7.8
Spleen-related benign diseases	196	64/132	37 ± 16	2.0 ± 0.4	13.4 ± 5.3
Immune thrombocytopenia	142	NR	NR	NR	NR
Spleen benign tumors	30	NR	NR	NR	NR
β-Thalassemia	11	NR	NR	NR	NR
Autoimmune hemolytic anemia	7	NR	NR	NR	NR
Hereditary spherocytosis	5	NR	NR	NR	NR
Niemann-Pick disease	1	NR	NR	NR	NR
Spleen-related malignant diseases	42	20/22	51 ± 17	2.5 ± 0.6	23.6 ± 8.7
Non-Hodgkin's lymphoma	30	NR	NR	NR	NR
Leukemia	8	NR	NR	NR	NR
Metastatic tumors	4	NR	NR	NR	NR
Splenomegaly and hypersplenism secondary to portal hypertension	64	29/35	47 ± 11	2.4 ± 0.6	22.6 ± 7.3

Note: NR means not reported

were completed in the subsequent 10 years. The surgical indications and main clinical symptoms of the patients are shown in Table 1.1 [19]. Immune thrombocytopenia, formerly as idiopathic thrombocytopenic purpura (ITP), accounted for nearly half (47%) of all diseases and more than 70% of spleen-related benign diseases in the patients. Non-Hodgkin's lymphoma (NHL) was the most common malignant disease. In addition, splenomegaly and hypersplenism secondary to portal hypertension constituted 21% of all diseases in the patients.

1.2.1 Hematological Disorders

In the early years, LS was most commonly performed for benign blood disorders complicated with normal-sized to mildly enlarged spleens such as ITP. The first meta-analysis on LS was published in 2003. The study analyzed 51 English papers with more than 20 cases between 1991 and 2002, including 26 controlled trials and sequence study of 25 cases. Of a total of 2119 patients, more than 80% were diagnosed with hematologic disorders, of which benign diseases accounted for 74.2% (ITP accounted for more than 70%) and malignant diseases, 9.5% (lymphoma accounted for more than 80%) [31].

With the better understanding of the role of spleen in immunity, anemia, and other hematologic disorders, as well as the improvements of diagnosis and treatment modalities, the indications for splenectomy are constantly expanding. At present, the common benign blood disorders requiring splenectomy include ITP, thrombotic thrombocytopenic purpura (TTP), hereditary spherocytosis (HS), autoimmune hemolytic anemia (AIHA), hemoglobinopathies (such as sickle cell anemia and thalassemia), and hemolytic anemia caused by erythrocyte enzyme deficiency (such as glucose-6-phosphate dehydrogenase, G6PD, deficiency, and pyruvate kinase deficiency). Some malignant blood disorders may also benefit from splenectomy, including Hodgkin's lymphoma, non-Hodgkin's lymphoma, hairy cell leukemia, chronic lymphocytic leukemia (CLL), and chronic myelogenous leukemia (CML).

Noteworthily, the decision on splenectomy for hematological disorders should be made by a multidisciplinary team dominated by hematologists.

1.2.2 Splenomegaly and Hypersplenism Secondary to Liver Cirrhosis and Portal Hypertension

Liver cirrhosis and portal hypertension always lead to congestive splenomegaly, hypersplenism and esophagogastric varices. Severe thrombocytopenia due to hypersplenism significantly increases the risk of spontaneous bleeding and complicates the diagnostic or therapeutic procedures such as liver biopsy and interferon therapy. Therefore, splenectomy and pericardial devascularization are still widely performed for patients with splenomegaly and hypersplenism secondary to liver cirrhosis and portal hypertension in Asian countries.

However, massive splenomegaly results in small operation space, and impaired coagulation and perigastric varices increase the risk of massive hemorrhage in operation. In 2008, splenomegaly and hypersplenism secondary to liver cirrhosis and portal hypertension were classified as contraindications for LS in the guideline of the European Association for Endoscopic Surgery (EAES). Thereafter, many authors from China and Japan attempted to study LS. In 2012, we conducted a systematic review to assess the safety and efficacy of LS for patients with liver cirrhosis and portal hypertension [13]. In recent years, five more systematic reviews and meta-analyses have been published [23, 32–35]. The main results are presented in Table 1.2. It is clear that the rate of conversion to laparotomy is about 5%, mostly due to uncontrollable massive bleeding. Although LS requires longer operation time than OS (averagely 30–40 min more), it has such advantages as significantly less blood loss (averagely 200–300 mL less), shorter length of postoperative hospital stay (averagely 3–5 days less), and similar or lower incidence of postoperative complications. In 2015, the guideline of Japan Society for Endoscopic Surgery (JSES) included liver cirrhosis and portal hypertension as indications for LS.

It is noteworthy that the above systematic reviews and meta-analyses were all from China, and most of the literatures included were also from China and Japan, which may reflect the significant difference in the understanding of the role of splenectomy in the treatment of hypersplenism secondary to liver cirrhosis and portal hypertension between the Eastern and Western counties. In Western countries, the incidence of severe thrombocytopenia in cirrhotic patients is relatively low, that is, platelet count is less than 40×10^9/L in only 1% of patients; on the contrary, the incidence of thrombosis in the portal venous system is relatively high after splenectomy [36]. Therefore, splenectomy is seldom performed. In Eastern countries, however, it is believed that splenectomy not only reverses thrombocytopenia but also improves liver function, immune status, and portal hypertensive gastropathy [13]. Our follow-up studies confirmed that laboratory indicators of blood system and liver function continued to improve after splenectomy [9, 16, 20]. Therefore, LS is safe and effective in the treatment of liver cirrhosis and portal hypertension.

1.2.3 Occupying Lesions of the Spleen

The occupying lesions of the spleen include benign diseases and malignant tumors. The common benign diseases are splenic cysts, splenic abscess, hemangioma, lymphangioma, and littoral cell angioma (LCA). The majority of the malignant lesions are metastatic tumors, with an incidence of about 7% in cancer patients. The common primary cancers are breast cancer, lung cancer, melanoma, nasopharyngeal cancer, etc. By contrast, the primary malignant tumor of the spleen is rare, which is commonly angiosarcoma or lymphangiosarcoma [37–39].

1.2.4 Spleen Injury

The application of LS in splenic rupture caused by trauma is limited, since patients with grades I–III damage and hemodynamic stability are treated with nonsurgical therapy and splenic vascular embolization when necessary, while patients with grades IV–V damage often undergo massive bleeding and hemodynamic instability, which make LS inapplicable [38]. We summarized indications for LS in long-term clinical practice, including (1) CT scan showing unipolar spleen injury without splenic pedicle injury, (2) blood pressure >90/60 mmHg and heart rate <120 bpm, and (3) no signs of multi-organ injury [27, 30].

Table 1.2 Systematic review and meta-analysis of laparoscopic splenectomy in patients with liver cirrhosis and portal hypertension

First author	Year of publication	Country	Databases retrieved	Starting and ending time of retrieval	No. of included studies	Interventions	No. of patients	Conversion [n (%)]	Operation time (min)	Blood loss (mL)	Postoperative hospital stay (days)	Complications (%)
Chen XD [13]	2013	China	PubMed, Embase	August 2012	16	LS	478	21 (4.4)	142–259	141–506	2.6–17.6	15.1
						OS	197	NA	135–205	109–750	10.1–19.4	17.3
						LSD	173	11 (6.4)	184–341	90–550	6.5–19.8	24.3
						OSD	124		178–230	350–1850	12.5–35.6	26.6
Zheng X [32]	2015	China	PubMed, Springerlink, ScienceDirect (Elsevier)	NR	8	LS + LSD	326	NR	224 (150–341)	191.2 (129.1–531)	8.2 (6.1–19.8)	37.1
						OS + OSD	399	NA	180 (135–234.5)	415.5 (100–778)	11.9 (10.1–35.6)	38.6
						Pooled data			MD = 35.24 [16.74, 53.74]; $Z = 3.73$; $P < 0.001$	MD = −194.84 [−321.34, −68.34]; $Z = 3.02$; $P = 0.003$	MD = −4.33 [−5.30, −3.36]; $Z = 8.79$; $P < 0.001$	OR = 0.74 [0.52, 1.06]; $Z = 1.63$; $P = 0.100$
Cai YQ [23]	2014	China	PubMed, Embase, MEDLINE	1991–2012	5	LS	180	9 (5)	194.1	214.8	7.7	22.7
						OS	243		171.2	568.3	13.02	30.9
Al-raimi K [34]	2016		PubMed, Springer, Cochrane Reviews, Ovid, Embase	June 2015	7	LS	232	NR	150–224	70.3–359	6.1–14.6	21.1
						OS	277	NA	100–205	109–750	8.8–19.4	27.1
		China				Pooled data			MD = 31.58 [9.82, 53.34]; $Z = 2.84$; $P = 0.004$	MD = −210.30 [−409.32, −11.28]; $Z = 2.07$; $P = 0.04$	MD = −3.41 [−4.43, −2.39]; $Z = 6.56$; $P < 0.00001$	OR = 0.75 [0.50, 1.14]; $Z = 1.38$; $P = 0.17$

Jiang GQ [33]	2015	China	PubMed	Dec 31, 2014	15	LSD	412	22 (5.4)	221.7	192.7	9.5	29.9
						OSD	200	NA	201.3	301.6	14.3	45.5
Yu HB [35]	2016		CCRCT, Medline, SCI, EMBASE, CNKI, Wanfang Database, CBD	July 2014	17	LSD	552	NR	190–336	90–1768	6.3–16.4	14.0
						OSD	541	NA	152–305	327–2412	8.4–22.7	29.5
		China				Pooled data			MD = 42.16 [32.20, 52.11]; $Z = 8.30$; $P < 0.00001$	MD = –330.62 [–552.35, –88.90]; $Z = 2.71$; $P = 0.007$	MD = –4.19 [–6.19, –2.19]; $Z = 4.10$; $P < 0.0001$	OR = 0.43 [0.29, 0.64]; $Z = 4.20$; $P < 0.0001$

Note: *CCRCT* Cochrane Central Register of Controlled Trials, *SCI* Science Citation Index, *CNKI* China National Knowledge Infrastructure, *CBD* China biomedical database, *LS* laparoscopic splenectomy, *LSD* laparoscopic splenectomy with devascularization, *OS* open splenectomy, *OSD* open splenectomy with devascularization, *NR* not reported, *NA* not applicable, *MD* mean difference, *OR* odds ratio

1.2.5 Miscellaneous

Other rare indications include the wandering spleen, systemic lupus erythematosus (SLE)-induced thrombocytopenia [17], Niemann-Pick disease [18], Gaucher disease, and other unexplained splenomegaly.

1.3 Contraindications

1.3.1 Absolute Contraindications

1. Severe medical comorbidities such as severe cardiopulmonary diseases.
2. Uncorrected coagulation dysfunction.
3. Intolerance to pneumoperitoneum.
4. Hemodynamically unstable splenic trauma.

1.3.2 Relative Contraindications

1.3.2.1 Supermassive Splenomegaly

Splenomegaly is common in benign and malignant blood disorders and portal hypertension. Mild to moderate splenomegaly does not significantly increase the difficulty of surgery. However, massive splenomegaly (longitudinal length >20 cm or spleen weight >1000 g), especially supermassive splenomegaly (longitudinal length >22 cm or spleen weight >1600 g), markedly increases the difficulty of operation, leading to high conversion rate. With advancement of instruments and improvement of surgical skills, especially the introduction of hand-assisted laparoscopic surgery and preoperative splenic artery embolization, spleen size is no longer a contraindicated factor of LS [1, 2].

1.3.2.2 Thrombocytopenia

Patients requiring splenectomy are often associated with thrombocytopenia, even very low platelets ($<10 \times 10^9$/L), and sometimes completely unresponsive to medical treatment or even platelet infusion. Splenectomy itself is the most effective treatment for thrombocytopenia, so platelet count is no longer contraindicated for these patients [40].

1.3.2.3 Morbid Obesity

Morbid obesity (BMI > 35 kg/m^2) leads to narrow operation space and difficulty in exposure. Although LS in these patients is associated with prolonged operation time, increased blood loss, and higher risk of conversion to laparotomy, it reduces postoperative complications, especially wound complications. Therefore, morbid obesity is not a contraindication for LS [41, 42].

1.3.2.4 Elderly

Age itself is not an obstacle to LS, but older patients are more likely associated with more comorbidities, worse ASA scores, increased postoperative complications, and longer postoperative hospital stay.

1.3.2.5 Pregnancy

Clinical evidence of LS in pregnant women is relatively lacking, and only a few cases have been reported. It should be carried out cautiously [1, 43–45].

1.4 Comparison Between LS and OS

1.4.1 Literatures

There are three meta-analyses comparing LS with OS, and their main characteristics are shown in Table 1.3 [31, 46, 47].

1.4.2 Results

The main results of the meta-analyses are shown in Table 1.4.

1.4.3 Conclusions

Although LS has a longer operation time than OS, LS is more advantageous for its significant reduction in intraoperative blood loss, blood transfusion, postoperative hospital stay, and incidences of morbidity and mortality.

Table 1.3 Systemic review and meta-analysis for comparison between LS and OS

First author	Year of publication	Country	Journal	Databases retrieved	Starting and ending time of retrieval	No. of included studies	No. of involved patients
Winslow ER [31]	2003	America	Surgery	Medline	January 1991 to December 2002	51 26 paired studies 25 unpaired studies	1697 (control studies) LS 876 OS 821
Chen J [46]	2014	China	Chin Med J	PubMed, Embase, Cochrane Library, Ovid, Web of Science	1990 to December 20, 2013	35 1 RCT 34 nonRCT	7269 LS 3981 OS 3288
Cheng J [47]	2016	China	Surg Endosc	PubMed, EMBASE, Web of Science, Cochrane Library	1999 to 2014	37 control studies	5035 LS 2909 OS 2126

Note: *CL* Cochrane library, *WOS* web of science, *LS* laparoscopic splenectomy, *OS* open splenectomy, *RCT* randomized controlled trial

1.4.4 Discussion

The three meta-analyses were included in the literatures of different periods comparing LS and OS, and basically consistent results were obtained, that is, LS is superior to OS. Winslow et al. [31] included the literatures in early period and focused on the analysis of postoperative complications. It was found that the rates of pulmonary, wound, infectious, and gastrointestinal complications were all significantly lower in the LS group than those of OS, especially the incidence of subphrenic abscess was very low (LS 0.1%) but occurred in 2.4% of patients in the OS group, whereas there was no significant difference in the rates of cardiac, thrombotic, neurologic, or urinary complications between the two groups. Chen et al. [46] included more literatures, involving markedly large sample size and all kinds of nontraumatic splenic diseases. Due to significant statistical heterogeneity ($I^2 > 90\%$) for numerical variables such as operation time, blood loss, and postoperative hospital stay across studies, the random effects model was used to pool the data, still showing advantages of LS; by contrast, there was no obvious heterogeneity for categorical variables such as transfusion rate, complication rate, and mortality, and the fixed effects method were applied and revealed reduced need for blood transfusion, postoperative morbidity, and mortality rates in LS. Cheng et al. [47] included more recent literatures in recent 15 years when LS was relatively well-developed. In particular, they carried out subgroup analysis according to different diseases, showing that LS was superior to OS in all diseases. Noteworthily, a significant change from the results of the previous two meta-analyses was that the operation time of LS is not significantly different from that of OS, indicating that the operation time of LS was significantly shortened with the improvement of surgical techniques and equipment. We compared LS with OS in the settings of hypersplenism secondary to liver cirrhosis and splenomegaly, respectively, and found similar results to the above meta-analyses (Table 1.5).

1.5 Hand-Assisted Laparoscopic Splenectomy (HALS)

1.5.1 Literatures

At present, there is only one systematic review and meta-analysis comparing HALS with traditional LS (CLS), which retrieved the English literature comparing HALS with CLS from three databases, i.e., "MEDLINE, EMBASE, Cochrane Library" up to September 2013. The study included nine non-randomized controlled studies involving 463 patients (170 with HALS and 293 with CLS) [48].

Table 1.4 Results of systemic review and meta-analysis for comparison between LS and OS

Study	Group	Operation time (min)	Blood loss (mL)	Rate of transfusion	Postoperative hospital stay (day)	Morbidity	Mortality
Winslow ER [31]	LS	1[illegible]9.9	224.9	10.2%	3.6	15.5%	0.6%
	OS	1[illegible]4.1	254.4	14.0%	7.2	26.6%	1.1%
	***P*-value**	<0.0001	NS	<0.02	<0.001	<0.0001	NS
Chen J [46]	Meta-analysis	$n = 21$; WMD = 42.65 [−5.58, 59.73]; $P < 0.00001$; $I^2 = 95\%$	$n = 12$; WMD = −133.95 [−229.02, −38.88]; $P = 0.006$; $I^2 = 97\%$	$n = 18$; OR = 0.53 [0.39, 0.72]; $P < 0.00001$; $I^2 = 39\%$	$n = 20$; WMD = −2.73 [−3.34, −2.12]; $P < 0.00001$; $I^2 = 88\%$	$n = 26$; OR = 0.44 [0.38, 0.51]; $P < 0.00001$; $I^2 = 20\%$	$n = 13$; LS: 1.38% vs. OS: 3.79%; OR = 0.38 [0.24, 0.59]; $P < 0.0001$; $I^2 = 0\%$
Cheng J [47]	Overall ($n = 11$)	WMD = 19.30 [−39.36, 77.96]; $P = 0.52$; $I^2 = 97\%$	WMD = −217.67 [−325.07, −110.27]; $P < 0.0001$; $I^2 = 99\%$	NR	WMD = −2.10 [−2.84, −1.36]; $P < 0.00001$; $I^2 = 92\%$	OR = 0.44 [0.36, 0.54]; $P < 0.00001$; $I^2 = 0\%$	OR = 0.87 [0.09, 8.43], $P = 0.90$; $I^2 = 56\%$
	Hematologic disorders ($n = 4$)	WMD = 0.66 [−69.02, 70.34]; $P = 0.99$; $I^2 = 95\%$	WMD = −102.47 [−152.65, −52.29]; $P < 0.0001$; $I^2 = 0\%$	NR	WMD = −2.15 [−2.68, −1.62]; $P < 0.00001$; $I^2 = 0\%$	OR = 0.36 [0.16, 0.84]; $P = 0.02$; $I^2 = 30\%$	NR
	Massive splenomegaly ($n = 5$)	WMD = 10.13 [−32.85, 53.10]; $P = 0.64$; $I^2 = 92\%$	WMD = −168.37 [−312.78, −23.96]; $P = 0.02$; $I^2 = 88\%$	NR	WMD = −4.14 [−5.58, −2.70]; $P < 0.00001$; $I^2 = 68\%$	OR = 0.53 [0.30–0.94]; $P = 0.03$; $I^2 = 0\%$	NR
	Idiopathic thrombocytopenic purpura ($n = 7$)	WMD = 13.59 [−38.51, 65.68]; $P = 0.61$; $I^2 = 99\%$	WMD = −174.30 [−284.74, −63.86]; $P = 0.002$; $I^2 = 95\%$	NR	WMD = −4.86 [−7.47, −2.26]; $P = 0.0003$; $I^2 = 96\%$	OR = 0.36 [0.18, 0.73]; $P = 0.005$; $I^2 = 52\%$	NR
	Children sickle cell disease ($n = 3$)	WMD = 49.33 [−37.86, 136.52]; $P = 0.27$; $I^2 = 96\%$	NR	NR	WMD = −1.68 [−2.47, −0.89]; $P < 0.0001$; $I^2 = 34\%$	OR = 0.20 [0.06, 0.69]; $P = 0.01$; $I^2 = 54\%$	NR
	Portal hypertension ($n = 7$)	WMD = 13.87 [−13.02, 40.75]; $P = 0.31$, $I^2 = 84\%$	WMD = −200.87 [−239.84, −161.89]; $P < 0.00001$; $I^2 = 84\%$	NR	WMD = −3.69 [−4.75, −2.63]; $P < 0.00001$, $I^2 = 67\%$	OR = 0.31 [0.19, 0.51]; $P < 0.00001$; $I^2 = 0\%$	NR

Note: *LS* laparoscopic splenectomy, *O[illegible]* open splenectomy, *NR* not reported, *WMD* weighted mean difference, *OR* odds ratio

Table 1.5 Comparison between LS and OS

Variable	Hypersplenism secondary to liver cirrhosis [6]			Massive splenomegaly (longitudinal length in CT scan > 20 cm) [5]		
	LS	OS	*P*-value	LS	OS	*P*-value
Patients	24	24		33	29	
Age (years)	50.5 ± 10.9	44.6 ± 13.7	NS	48.2 ± 14.8	44.5 ± 13.0	NS
Sex (M/F)	10/14	13/11	NS	17/16	16/13	NS
Diagnosis						
Liver cirrhosis	24	24		22	28	
Mediterranean disease	0	0		7	0	
Hereditary spherocytosis	0	0		2	0	
Lymphoma	0	0		2	1	
Conversion to OS	1	NA		1	NA	
Operation time (min)	224 ± 44	186 ± 83	NS	219.9 ± 43.4	182.3 ± 66.8	0.011
Blood loss (mL)	162 ± 126	421 ± 347	0.021	163.0 ± 56.2	420.9 ± 177.3	0.000
Spleen weight (g)	1405 ± 752	1243 ± 418	NS	1450.8 ± 345.7	1554.6 ± 283.8	NS
Transfusion	2 (8.3%)	9 (37.5%)	0.016	5 (15.1%)	15 (51.7%)	0.003
Hospital stay (days)	7.5 ± 1.7	9.9 ± 3.4	0.014	7.5 ± 1.7	10.1 ± 2.4	<0.001
Analgesia (cases)	4 (16.7)	14 (58.3)	0.003	NR	NR	NR
Oral intake (days)	1.6 ± 1	3.2 ± 0.9	0	NR	NR	NR
Complications (cases)	3 (12.5%)	10 (41.7%)	0.028	3 (9.1%)	10 (34.5%)	0.026

Note: *LS* laparoscopic splenectomy, *OS* open splenectomy, *M* male, *F* female, *NS* not significant, *NR* not reported, *NA* not applicable

1.5.2 Results

Even though spleen weight was heavier in the HALS group (CLS vs. HALS WMD = −0.93 kg; 95% CI: −1.74 to −0.11; P = 0.03; I^2 = 90%), the rate of conversion to laparotomy was significantly higher in the CLS group than that of HALS (CLS 26/290 vs. HALS 7/166; OR = 2.98; 95% CI: 1.28–6.93; P = 0.01; I^2 = 23%). Meanwhile, there was no difference with regard to operation time, blood loss, blood transfusion, intraoperative complications, postoperative hospital stay, and incidence of morbidity and mortality.

1.5.3 Conclusions

HALS was superior to CLS in patients with massive splenomegaly, which needs to be confirmed by randomized trials.

1.5.4 Discussion

HALS was first introduced by Kusminsky et al. [49] in 1995. In the setting of splenomegaly, HALS has the advantages of shortening the learning curve, facilitating the control of massive bleeding, and reducing conversion to open surgery. In 2012, we compared HALS (n = 19) with CLS (n = 20) [11] in patients with splenomegaly due to liver cirrhosis (massive splenomegaly, longitudinal length >17 cm; supermassive splenomegaly, longitudinal length >22 cm), and the results showed that HALS significantly reduced operation time (124 ± 42 min vs. 195 ± 43 min, P = 0) and blood loss (92 ± 65 mL vs. 169 ± 136 mL, P = 0.031) and transfusion (5% vs. 20%), and the subgroup analysis showed that HALS is more advantageous for supermassive splenomegaly. Moreover, HALS does not prolong the length of hospital stay (7.2 ± 2.8 days vs. 8.5 ± 2.3 days) nor increase

Table 1.6 Comparison between HALS and LS in complicated splenectomy

	HALS	LS	*P*-value
Patients	41	45	
Age (years)	50 ± 14	48 ± 13	NS
Sex (M/F)	22/19	23/22	NS
Spleen size (cm)	27.4 ± 7.6	24.7 ± 5.1	0.041
Diagnosis			NS
Portal hypertension	21 (51.2%)	27 (60%)	
Supramassive splenomegaly (>22 cm)	20 (48.8%)	18 (40%)	
Non-Hodgkin's lymphoma	14	11	
Leukemia	0	1	
β-Thalassemia	3	3	
Autoimmune hemolytic anemia	0	1	
Niemann-Pick disease	0	1	
Hereditary spherocytosis	1	1	
Splenomegaly of unknown origin	2	0	
Operation time (min)	136 ± 41	179 ± 54	<0.001
Blood loss (mL)	81 ± 57	149 ± 84	<0.001
Intraoperative transfusion (*n*)	3 (7.3%)	9 (20.0%)	NS
Conversion to OS (*n*)	0	2 (4.5%)	NS
Analgesia (*n*)	12 (26.8%)	6 (13.0%)	NS
Complications (cases)	17 (41.5%)	22 (49.0%)	NS
Time to full diet (days)	2.1 ± 0.9	2.3 ± 0.9	NS
Postoperative stay (days)	8.5 ± 2.9	8.8 ± 3.5	NS
Mortality [*n* (%)]	1 (2.4%)	0	NS

Note: *HALS* hand-assisted laparoscopic splenectomy, *LS* laparoscopic splenectomy, *NS* not significant

postoperative complication rate (21% vs. 45%). Therefore, we concluded that HALS is a better choice for patients with supermassive splenomegaly complicated with liver cirrhosis. In 2013, we included additional patients with supermassive splenomegaly due to other reasons for further analysis, which further verified our previous conclusion (Table 1.6) [18].

1.6 Single-Incision Laparoscopic Splenectomy (SILS)

1.6.1 Literatures

Four literatures introduce a systematic review or meta-analysis on SILS. The literatures by Targarona et al. [50], Fan et al. [51], and Gkegkes et al. [52] were systematic reviews, which included case reports and case series, without meta-analysis. Wu et al. [53] included 10 retrospective comparative studies for meta-analysis, involving 332 patients, of whom 146 underwent SILS and 186 CLS.

1.6.2 Results

Statistical analyses of the pooled estimates showed no significant difference between SILS and CLS, with regard to operation time (WMD = 13.17, 95% CI: 9.43–35.76, $P = 0.253$, $I^2 = 89.0\%$), blood loss (WMD = –1.57, 95% CI: –25.41–22.27, $P = 0.897$, $I^2 = 77.4\%$), conversion rate (OR = 1.81, 95% CI: 0.71–4.63, $P = 0.212$, $I^2 = 7.5\%$), postoperative hospital stay (WMD = –0.08 95% CI: –0.47–0.31, $P = 0.686$, $I^2 = 0.0\%$), total complication rate (OR = 0.97, 95% CI: 0.47–2.00; $P = 0.934$, $I^2 = 0.0\%$), starting time of feeding (WMD = 0.16, 95% CI: –0.35–0.67, $P = 0.534$, $I^2 = 54.9\%$), analgesics usage (WMD = –1.01, 95% CI: –7.58–5.56, $P = 0.763$; $I^2 = 0.0\%$), or pain score (WMD = –1.29, 95% CI: –3.06–0.47, $P = 0.151$; $I^2 = 94.7\%$) [53].

1.6.3 Conclusions

SILS is safe and feasible, but has no significant advantage over CLS.

1.6.4 Discussion

The application of SILS in the spleen is still in the beginning stage and was first reported by Barbaros et al. [54] in 2009. At present, there are few studies on SILS, and most of them are case reports or small sample-sized case series. Although it is a more technically demanding and challenging procedure, SILS is safe and feasible, without significantly prolonging the operation time or increasing blood loss, conversion to laparotomy, as well as complication rates. On the other hand, SILS does not show significant advantages in postoperative recovery, alleviating pain, or cosmetic effects. In light of the absence of high-quality clinical evidence, skilled surgeons can perform SILS cautiously to obtain more clinical data.

1.7 Robotic Splenectomy (RS)

1.7.1 Literatures

At present, there is no systematic review or meta-analysis on RS. There are three retrospective studies comparing RS with CLS, involving 391 patients, 128 of whom received RS and 263 CLS [55–57]. Giza et al. [57] assigned the patients to a simple splenectomy group or difficult splenectomy group according to the degree of surgical complexity.

1.7.2 Results

The main results were presented in Table 1.7. In the comparisons of patients from the easy groups reported by Bodner et al., Gelmini et al., and Giza et al., there was no significant difference in operation time, blood loss, conversion rate, postoperative hospital stay, and complication rate between RS and CLS. In the difficult splenectomy group of Giza, however, RS was associated with shorter operation time, less blood loss, lower conversion rate, and higher therapeutic success than CLS. In addition, both Bodner and Gelmini reported that the cost of RS was significantly higher than that of CLS ($P < 0.05$).

1.7.3 Conclusions

RS was safe and feasible, but showed a great challenge in techniques, so it should be performed by experienced surgeons.

1.7.4 Discussion

RS has some benefits (e.g., availability of three-dimensional vision, greater dexterity with instruments), which may save the surgeon's physical strength, eliminate hand tremors, and allow more meticulous dissection. Unfortunately, the high cost of equipment and instruments limits its widespread use.

1.8 Laparoscopic Partial Splenectomy (LPS)

1.8.1 Literatures

There is only one systematic review on LPS. The author searched the MEDLINE (PubMed) database by March 31, 2014, and included 33 literatures, all of which were case reports, case series, and retrospective cohort studies, involving 187 patients (168 patients with conventional LPS, 1 patient with single-incision LPS, and 18 patients with robotic LPS) [58].

1.8.2 Results

Most of the patients were children and young adults, aged from 6 to 58 years, with a median of 21 years. The most common indication is hereditary spherocytosis ($n = 97$, 52%), followed

Table 1.7 Comparison between RS and LS

	Bodner J 2005 [55]			Gelmini R 2011 [56]			Giza DE 2014 [57] Easy group (MISS < 3)			Giza DE 2014 [57] Difficult group (MISS ≥ 3)		
	LS	RS	*P*-value	LS	RS	*P*-value	LS	RS	*P*-value	LS	RS	*P*-value
Patients	6	6		45	45		141	23		71	54	
Sex (M/F)	0/6	2/4	NS	24/21	28/17	NR	NR	NR	NR	NR	NR	NR
Age (years)	62	42	NS	45.9	41	NR	NR	NR	NR	NR	NR	NR
BMI (kg/m^2)	26.3	27	NS	NR	NR	NR	NR	NR	NR	NR	NR	NR
ASA score	3	2	NS	NR	NR	NR	NR	NR	NR	NR	NR	NR
Spleen size	NR	NR	NR	15	13	NR	NR	NR	NR	NR	NR	NR
Operation time (min)	154 (115–29[illegible]	127 (95–174)	NS	125	153	<0.05	66.62 (23.14)	63.04 (17.40)	0.532	97.2 (24.57)	84.13 (24.1)	0.004
Blood loss (mL)	NR	NR	NR	NR	NR	NR	34.02 (17.16)	25.82 (11.53)	0.316	156.9 (67.3)	30.88 (12.1)	<0.001
Conversion rate	0	0	NS	5 (11.1%)	4 (8.9%)	NS	7 (5%)	0 (0%)	0.340	4 (5.6%)	0 (0%)	0.036
Transfusion rate	NR	NR	NR	0	0	NS	NR	NR	NR	NR	NR	NR
Postoperative stay (days)	7 (5–11)	6 (4–7)	NS	5.3	5.1	NS	NR	NR	NR	NR	NR	NR
Postoperative complication [n (%)]	0	0	NS	5 (11.1%)	5 (11.1%)	NS	2 (1.4%)	0 (0%)	0.738	2 (2.8%)	1 (1.9%)	0.602
Postoperative food intake (days)	NR	NR	NR	2.5	2.7	NS	NR	NR	NR	NR	NR	NR
Therapeutic success	NR	NR	NR	NR	NR	NR	135 (96%)	23 (100%)	0.398	64 (90%)	54 (100%)	0.017
Costs (US$)	4084	6927	<0.05	2590	6930	<0.05	NR	NR	NR	NR	NR	NR

Notes: *LS* laparoscopic splenectomy, *RS* robotic splenectomy, *CLS* conventional laparoscopic splenectomy, *MISS* Minimally Invasive Splenectomy Score, *NR* not reported, *NS* not significant by non-parasitic cysts (n = 46, 25%) and vascular malformations such as hemangioma, hemolymphangioma, and hamartoma (n = 13, 7%), and other rare indications included parasitic cysts (n = 4, 2%), metastatic tumor, abscess, laceration, hematoma, aneurysm, and so on. Two patients (1.1%) were converted to open surgery due to uncontrollable massive bleeding, but all patients successfully preserved part of their spleens. Most authors described blood loss as "minimal," occasionally reaching 300–450 mL. Only five patients (2.98%) received blood transfusion. The operation time ranged from 70 to 216 min and was relatively shorter (108–120 min) in the robotic LPS. The postoperative hospital stay was 1–8 days, with a median of 4 days. The incidence of surgical complications was low (n = 9, 5.36%), and there were no severe postoperative complications. It was noteworthy that three patients developed ischemia of residual spleen, and all of them successfully received conservative treatment.

1.8.3 Conclusions

Although LPS is safe and feasible, it is definitely a highly technically demanding and challenging procedure, which should be only performed by experienced surgeons in selected centers.

1.8.4 Discussion

The spleen is the largest immune organ of the body, which plays an important role in anti-infection. The overwhelming post splenectomy infection (OPSI) has always been one of the focused issues in splenic surgery. In the middle of the twentieth century, therefore, some scholars proposed partial splenectomy, which gradually gained general recognition [59, 60]. LPS was first performed by Poulin et al. [61] in 1995 for a trauma patient. With the continuous development of laparoscopic splenic surgery, LPS is not only increasingly performed in elective surgery, but also applied in emergency setting.

From 2011 to 2013, we performed LPS for 11 patients aged from 13 to 57 (median age 33, average 33.9 ± 16.1). The indications included non-parasitic cyst (n = 6), lymphangioma (n = 3), and hemangioma (n = 2), with the diameter of splenic lesions ranging from 4 to 9.5 cm, median 5 cm, and average 5.3 ± 1.6 cm. In terms of location, seven cases had their lesions on the upper spleen and four on the lower spleen. The mean operation time was 148 min (110–200 min). The mean estimated blood loss was 189 mL (100–400 mL). One patient was converted to total splenectomy because of hemorrhaging. Two patients suffered from postoperative complications: one who was converted to total splenectomy suffered from portal vein thrombosis, and the other who underwent partial splenectomy suffered from fluid collection around splenic recess. There was no blood transfusion and postoperative mortality. All patients were discharged uneventfully 5 days (4–7 days) after surgery. The postoperative follow-up after 6 months showed that the quality of life (SF-36 questionnaire) of the patients were the same as normal people. CT scan showed the volume of residual spleen increased by 15% (5–22%) [26].

On the favorable basis of elective LPS, we attempted to carry out LPS in emergency patients with traumatic splenic rupture from 2013. The selection criteria for emergency LPS were as follows: (1) preoperative CT scan that revealed single pole rupture without spleen pedicle injury; (2) BP > 90/60 mmHg and heart rates <120 bpm; and (3) no sign of multiple organ injury [30]. The results showed that LPS was safe and feasible in an emergency setting of traumatic splenic rupture (Table 1.8).

1.9 Laparoscopic Splenectomy in Children

1.9.1 Literatures

There is only one systematic review on LS in children, which retrieved the literatures comparing LS with OS among children in three databases, i.e., "MEDLINE, EMBASE and Web of Science" from 1993 to 2015. Ten comparative studies involved 922 patients, with 508 receiving LS and 414 receiving CLS [62].

Table 1.8 Comparison between LPS and LS in an emergency setting of traumatic splenic rupture

	LPS ($n = 21$)	LS ($n = 20$)	P-value
Sex (M/F)	16/5	16/4	0.874
Age (years)	36.0 ± 9.7	35.5 ± 9.9	0.917
Cause of splenic rupture			0.813
Traffic accident	13	14	
Blunt injury	6	4	
High falling	2	2	
Splenic size (cm)	14.2 ± 1.8 (12–17)	13.9 ± 1.6 (12–16.5)	0.882
Remnant part size (cm)	5.5 ± 1.2	NA	NA
Rupture site Upper pole (n)	12/21 (57.1%)	8/20 (40%)	0.272
Operation time (min)	122.6 ± 17.2	110.5 ± 18.7	0.117
Blood loss (mL)	174 ± 22	169 ± 29	0.331
Autologous transfusion (mL)	221 ± 36	206 ± 27	0.078
Allogeneic transfusion (mL)	125 ± 25	150 ± 30	0.878
Conversion (n)	0	0	1.000
Complications (n)	4 (19.0%)	4 (20.0%)	0.731
Length of hospital stay (days)	5.2 ± 1.1	4.9 ± 1.3	0.768
Late infection (n)	0% (0/21)	3 (15.0%)	0.107
Platelets count	$147 \pm 48 \times 10^9$/L	$282 \pm 61 \times 10^9$/L	0.031
Leukocyte count	$6.7 \pm 1.1 \times 10^9$/L	$8.9 \pm 1.9 \times 10^9$/L	0.017

Notes: *LPS* laparoscopic partial splenectomy, *LS* laparoscopic splenectomy, *M* male, *F* female, *NA* not applicable

1.9.2 Results

Meta-analysis showed that there was longer operation time (WMD = 42.22, 95% CI: 7.69–76.74; $P = 0.02$; $I^2 = 99\%$) while less blood loss (WMD = –31.77, 95% CI: –59.74–3.8; $P = 0.03$; $I^2 = 98\%$) and shorter length of hospital stay (WMD = –1.61, 95% CI: –2.19–1.02; $P = 0.001$; $I^2 = 87\%$) with the LS approach compared with OS. However, no significant difference was found between LS and OS in the secondary outcome, such as the removal of accessory spleens or total postoperative complications (LS: $n = 48$, 9.4% vs. OS: $n = 72$, 17.4%; WMD = 1.13, 95% CI: 0.68–1.89; $P = 0.64$; $I^2 = 0\%$), including postoperative high fever, acute chest syndrome, and ileus.

1.9.3 Conclusions

LS is a feasible, safe, and effective surgical procedure alternative to OS for pediatric patients, offering some advantages of less blood loss, shorter hospital stay, and relatively lower total postoperative complications.

1.9.4 Discussion

Compared with adults, pediatric patients have special anatomical and physiological characteristics. The most common indications for splenectomy in children are hereditary spherocytosis, chronic ITP, sickle cell anemia, and β-thalassemia, in which splenomegaly is more common. Meanwhile, the abdominal cavity is narrow in children, which significantly increases the difficulty of maneuvers, and leads to greater possibility of conversion to laparotomy. A child's immune system is underdeveloped, increasing the risk of infection complications, especially OPSI. Therefore, it is suggested that splenectomy should be postponed after 6 years old as far as possible. If possible, partial splenectomy may be alternatively considered. Besides, prophylactic vaccination for *Streptococcus pneumoniae*,

Neisseria meningitidis, and *Haemophilus influenzae* type B is recommended.

1.10 Portal Venous Thrombosis After Laparoscopic Splenectomy

Portal venous thrombosis (PVT) is a special complication after splenectomy, and its clinical manifestations are relatively insidious. Most patients may have no symptoms or mild non-specific symptoms, but a few patients may have fatal intestinal necrosis. Therefore, sufficient attention should be paid to it.

The incidence of PVT after LS varies widely across studies, but many scholars believe that it may be underestimated (Table 1.9) [63–84]. The reported incidence ranged from 2.6% to 78.6%, with a mean of 24.8% (SD 22.6%, 95% CI 14.7%–34.8%) and a median of 19.2% (quartile 5.1%–41.1%). In subgroup analyses, the incidence of PVT seems higher in literatures after 2010, in prospective studies, in literatures using computed tomography (CT), in literatures with sample size ≥40, and in adults than that in literatures before 2010, in retrospective studies, in literatures using ultrasonography (USG), in literatures with sample size <40, and in children, respectively, although there were no statistically significant differences. However, the incidence was significantly higher in the Chinese and Japanese literatures and in patients with liver cirrhosis than that in the Western literatures and in non-cirrhotic patients, respectively (Table 1.10). Noteworthily, all studies in patients with liver cirrhosis were performed in China or Japan, and only two of the seven Eastern literatures studied non-cirrhotic patients. Actually, there was no significant difference between the patients with liver cirrhosis (47.5 ± 23.4) % and those without liver cirrhosis (52.0 ± 0.7) % in the Eastern literatures ($P = 0.809$).

The risk factors for PVT after LS are complex, involving anatomical (such as the size of the spleen, diameter of the splenic vein or portal vein), physiological (age, anticoagulant activity, liver function), disease (malignant tumor, cirrhosis), and surgical (surgical approach, operation time) factors. Fifteen studies analyzed the potential risk factors using case-control method, including spleen weight [63, 64, 66, 69, 70, 72, 76, 80], spleen size [71, 79, 80], operation time [78, 81, 82], diameter of splenic vein [70, 75], diameter of portal vein [78, 81], activity of antithrombin III [72], ICG R-15 (%) [75], total bilirubin [75], lupus anticoagulant [71], and intraoperative blood transfusion [79]. Although no randomized controlled trials or prospective studies compared the incidence of PVT between LS and OS, the results of three case-control studies suggested that the incidence of PVT after LS and OS was basically comparable [63, 73, 82].

In general, about half of the patients were asymptomatic (asymptomatic 118 vs. symptomatic 98). The reported asymptomatic rates ranged widely from 0% to 100%, with a mean of 43.7% (SD 36.9%, 95% CI 25.3%–62.0%) and a median of 47.5% (quartile 0%–76.8%). The most common symptoms included abdominal pain, fever, loss of appetite, nausea, and vomiting. If there was intestinal necrosis, there might be obvious signs of peritonitis. Laboratory examination usually found elevated white blood cells. Both enhanced CT and color Doppler ultrasound are highly sensitive detection techniques. The timing of examination in most studies was about 1 week after surgery. Once PVT is diagnosed, anticoagulant therapy should be initiated, usually with subcutaneous injection of low molecular weight heparin (LMWH) and oral administration of warfarin for at least 3 months and thrombus remission in most patients [68]. For patients with obvious signs of peritonitis and suspicion of intestinal necrosis, an emergency exploratory laparoscopy or laparotomy should be considered [63, 85].

An RCT with a small sample size ($n = 29$) studied whether the use of LMWH in patients with blood disorders for 21 days after LS reduced the incidence of PVT. The trial found that the incidence of PVT after LS was very low and it

Table 1.9 Studies on portal venous thrombosis after laparoscopic splenectomy

Investigator	Design	Country	Indication	Examination technique	Age	No. of patients	No. of PVT	Incidence (%)	No. of symptomatic patients	No. of asymptomatic patients
Winslow 2002 [63]	Retrospective	America	Non-cirrhosis	CT	Adult	35	2	5.7	2	0
Pietrabissa 2004 [64]	Prospective	Italy	Non-cirrhosis	USG	Adult	40	9	22.5	6	3
Harris 2005 [65]	Prospective	Canada	Non-cirrhosis	USG	Adult	14	2	14.3	0	2
Romano 2006 [66]	Prospective	Italy	Non-cirrhosis	USG	Adult	38	7	18.4	4	3
Ruiz-Tovar 2006 [67]	Prospective	Spain	Non-cirrhosis	CT	Adult	20	2	10.0	1	1
Svensson 2006 [68]	Retrospective	Sweden	Non-cirrhosis	CT	Adult	39	1	2.6	1	0
Ikeda 2007 [69]	Prospective	Japan	Non-cirrhosis	CT	Adult	33	17	51.5	4	13
Danno 2009 [70]	Prospective	Japan	Non-cirrhosis	CT	Adult	40	21	52.5	2	19
Tran 2010 [71]	Retrospective	Canada	Non-cirrhosis	USG	Adult	40	9	22.5	2	7
Kawanaka 2010 [72]	Prospective	Japan	Cirrhosis	CT	Adult	50	10	20.0	NR	NR
Vecchio 2011 [73]	Retrospective	Italy	Non-cirrhosis	USG	Adult	103	3	2.9	3	0
Wang 2011 [74]	Prospective	Canada	Non-cirrhosis	USG	Adult	29	1	3.4	0	1
Kakinoki 2012 [75]	Prospective	Japan	Cirrhosis	CT	Adult	28	22	78.6	12	10
Alexakis 2013 [76]	Prospective	Greece	Non-cirrhosis	USG	Adult	48	4	8.3	2	2
Cheng 2015 [77]	Retrospective	China	Cirrhosis	USG	Adult	219	82	37.4	NR	NR
Jiang 2016 [78]	Retrospective	China	Cirrhosis	USG	Adult	75	48	64.0	NR	NR
Manouchehri 2016 [79]	Prospective	Canada	Non-cirrhosis	USG	Adult	68	17	25.0	5	12
de'Angelis 2017 [80]	Prospective	France	Non-cirrhosis	CT	Adult	170	91	53.5	46	45
Qian 2017 [81]	Retrospective	China	Cirrhosis	CT	Adult	130	49	37.7	NR	NR
Rottenstreich 2017 [82]	Retrospective	Israel	Non-cirrhosis	CT	Adult	98	5	5.1	5	0
Oomen 2013 [83]	Retrospective	Nederland	Non-cirrhosis	USG	Child	40	2	5.0	2	0
Gelas 2014 [84]	Retrospective	France	Non-cirrhosis	USG	Child	26	1	3.8	1	0

Table 1.10 Subgroup analysis of incidence of portal venous thrombosis after laparoscopic splenectomy

	Sub-group	No. of studies	Mean	SD	*P*-value
Publishing era	Before 2010	10	22.0	17.2	0.613
	After 2010	12	27.1	26.9	
Study design	Retrospective	10	18.7	21.2	0.259
	Prospective	12	29.8	23.4	
Country	China/Japan	7	48.8	19.2	<0.001
	West countries	15	13.5	13.6	
Indication	Cirrhosis	5	47.5	23.4	0.007
	Non-cirrhosis	17	18.1	18.0	
Detection methods	USG	12	19.0	17.8	0.195
	CT	10	31.7	26.6	
Patients	≥40	13	27.4	20.3	0.521
	<40	9	20.9	26.4	
Age group	Child	2	4.4	0.8	0.189
	Adult	20	26.8	22.8	

was difficult to make a definite conclusion due to its small sample size [74]. Another two studies from Japan and China have shown that use of prophylactic anticoagulation (antithrombin III concentrate [72], LMWH, aspirin, or warfarin [81]) in patients with liver cirrhosis significantly reduced the incidence of PVT. In addition, in patients with cirrhosis, early postoperative use of LMWH was superior to low molecular dextran [77] and warfarin to aspirin [78]. Therefore, the use of LMWH for 1 week in the early postoperative period and oral warfarin up to 1 year after surgery in patients with liver cirrhosis may be effective in preventing PVT after LS.

1.11 Prospects

The superiority of LS over OS has been universally recognized. LS not only significantly reduces intraoperative blood loss, transfusion, and the rate of complications, but also accelerates postoperative recovery and shortens the length of hospital stay. As a result, it has been widely accepted as the "standard procedure" for splenectomy. However, patients needing splenectomy are usually complicated with other complex clinical conditions such as splenomegaly, severe thrombocytopenia, anemia, blood malignancies, liver cirrhosis, and portal hypertension, which make the procedure more difficult and technically demanding, limiting the widespread application of LS, especially in primary hospitals. The introduction of HALS has basically overcome the limitation caused by splenomegaly, and it is worth promoting its application in patients with massive splenomegaly.

Robot-assisted surgery is in the ascendant in developed countries in Europe and the United States, whereas only performed in a few medical centers in China. RS has the advantages in terms of better three-dimensional surgical vision, greater flexibility of instruments, and saving surgeons' physical energy. Nonetheless, much higher cost of equipment and instruments limits its universality. In the future, RS may play a greater role with the development of social economy and the reduction in the cost.

At present, the level of clinical evidence on LS is generally low. There are no more than ten RCTs, and most studies included in systematic reviews and meta-analyses are retrospective or non-randomized comparative studies. There are a large number of clinical problems needing further research, such as:

1. The long-term effects after LPS: can LPS improve the patient's immune status and effectively prevent OPSI?
2. The rational and effective detection method and timing of PVT, the prophylactic measures and duration of PVT, whether asymptomatic PVT needs treatment, the treatment method and duration of PVT.

3. What are the underlying reasons for difference in the treatment of splenectomy for patients with hypersplenism secondary to liver cirrhosis and portal hypertension between the East and the West? What is the long-term efficacy of LS in cirrhotic patients? Can LS improve the quality of life or prolong survival time? It is important to further clarify the value of LS, especially in our country, since LS is more commonly performed for cirrhotic patients.

References

1. Habermalz B, Sauerland S, Decker G, et al. Laparoscopic splenectomy: the clinical practice guidelines of the European Association for Endoscopic Surgery (EAES). Surg Endosc. 2008;22(4):821–48.
2. Tanaka M, Tomikawa M, Nakamura M, et al. General gastroenterological surgery: spleen. Asian J Endosc Surg. 2015;8(3):242–5.
3. Delaitre B, Maignien B. Splenectomy by the laparoscopic approach. Report of a case. [Article in French]. Presse Med. 1991;20(44):2263.
4. Chen X, Peng B, Cai Y, et al. Laparoscopic splenectomy for patients with immune thrombocytopenia and very low platelet count: is platelet transfusion necessary? J Surg Res. 2011;170(2):e225–32.
5. Zhou J, Wu Z, Cai Y, et al. The feasibility and safety of laparoscopic splenectomy for massive splenomegaly: a comparative study. J Surg Res. 2011;171(1):e55–60.
6. Cai YQ, Zhou J, Chen XD, et al. Laparoscopic splenectomy is an effective and safe intervention for hypersplenism secondary to liver cirrhosis. Surg Endosc. 2011;25(12):3791–7.
7. Wu Z, Zhou J, Pankaj P, et al. Laparoscopic splenectomy for immune thrombocytopenia (ITP) patients with platelet counts lower than 1 × 10^9/L. Int J Hematol. 2011;94(6):533–8.
8. Wu Z, Zhou J, Pankaj P, et al. Comparative treatment and literature review for laparoscopic splenectomy alone versus preoperative splenic artery embolization splenectomy. Surg Endosc. 2012;26(10):2758–66.
9. Zhou J, Wu Z, Pankaj P, et al. Long-term postoperative outcomes of hypersplenism: laparoscopic versus open splenectomy secondary to liver cirrhosis. Surg Endosc. 2012;26(12):3391–400.
10. Wu Z, Zhou J, Pankaj P, et al. Laparoscopic and open splenectomy for splenomegaly secondary to liver cirrhosis: an assessment of immunity. Surg Endosc. 2012;26(12):3557–64.
11. Wang X, Li Y, Zhou J, et al. Hand-assisted laparoscopic splenectomy is a better choice for patients with supramassive splenomegaly due to liver cirrhosis. J Laparoendosc Adv Surg Tech A. 2012;22(10):962–7.
12. Wu Z, Zhou J, Cai YQ, et al. The learning curve for laparoscopic splenectomy for massive splenomegaly: a single surgeon's experience. Chin Med J. 2013;126(11):2103–8.
13. Chen XD, He FQ, Yang L, et al. Laparoscopic splenectomy with or without devascularization of the stomach for liver cirrhosis and portal hypertension: a systematic review. ANZ J Surg. 2013;83(3):122–8.
14. Wang M, Zhang M, Zhou J, et al. Predictive factors associated with long-term effects of laparoscopic splenectomy for chronic immune thrombocytopenia. Int J Hematol. 2013;97(5):610–6.
15. Wu Z, Zhou J, Wang X, et al. Laparoscopic splenectomy for treatment of splenic marginal zone lymphoma. World J Gastroenterol. 2013;19(24):3854–60.
16. Zhou J, Wu Z, Wu J, et al. Transjugular intrahepatic portosystemic shunt (TIPS) versus laparoscopic splenectomy (LS) plus preoperative endoscopic varices ligation (EVL) in the treatment of recurrent variceal bleeding. Surg Endosc. 2013;27(8):2712–20.
17. Zhou J, Wu Z, Zhou Z, et al. Efficacy and safety of laparoscopic splenectomy in thrombocytopenia secondary to systemic lupus erythematosus. Clin Rheumatol. 2013;32(8):1131–8.
18. Wang X, Li Y, Peng B. Hand-assisted laparoscopic technique in the setting of complicated splenectomy: a 9-year experience. World J Surg. 2013;37(9):2046–52.
19. Wang X, Li Y, Crook N, et al. Laparoscopic splenectomy: a surgeon's experience of 302 patients with analysis of postoperative complications. Surg Endosc. 2013;27(10):3564–71.
20. Zhou J, Wu Z, Wu J, et al. Laparoscopic splenectomy plus preoperative endoscopic variceal ligation versus splenectomy with pericardial devascularization (Hassab's operation) for control of severe varices due to portal hypertension. Surg Endosc. 2013;27(11):4371–7.
21. Wang M, Zhang M, Li J, et al. Risk factors of portal vein thrombosis in patients with beta thalassemia major after splenectomy: laparoscopic versus open procedure. Hepato-Gastroenterology. 2014;61(129):48–54.
22. Wang MJ, Li JL, Zhou J, et al. Consecutive laparoscopic gallbladder and spleen resections in cirrhotic patients. World J Gastroenterol. 2014;20(2):546–54.
23. Cai Y, Liu Z, Liu X. Laparoscopic versus open splenectomy for portal hypertension: a systematic review of comparative studies. Surg Innov. 2014;21(4):442–7.
24. Cai Y, Liu X, Peng B. Should we routinely transfuse platelet for immune thrombocytopenia patients with platelet count less than 10 × 10^9/L who underwent laparoscopic splenectomy? World J Surg. 2014;38(9):2267–72.
25. Cai Y, Liu X, Peng B. A novel method for laparoscopic splenectomy in the setting of hypersplenism secondary to liver cirrhosis: ten years' experience. World J Surg. 2014;38(11):2934–9.

26. Wang X, Wang M, Zhang H, et al. Laparoscopic partial splenectomy is safe and effective in patients with focal benign splenic lesion. Surg Endosc. 2014;28(12):3273–8.
27. Cai YQ, Li CL, Zhang H, et al. Emergency laparoscopic partial splenectomy for ruptured spleen: a case report. World J Gastroenterol. 2014;20(46):17670–3.
28. Cai YQ, Wang X, Ran X, et al. Laparoscopic splenectomy for splenic littoral cell angioma. World J Gastroenterol. 2015;21(21):6660–4.
29. Wang M, Wei A, Zhang Z, et al. Laparoscopic splenectomy for the elderly liver cirrhotic patients with hypersplenism: a retrospective comparable study. Medicine (Baltimore). 2016;95(10):e3012.
30. Li H, Wei Y, Peng B, et al. Feasibility and safety of emergency laparoscopic partial splenectomy: a retrospective analysis. Medicine (Baltimore). 2017;96(16):e6450.
31. Winslow ER, Brunt LM. Perioperative outcomes of laparoscopic versus open splenectomy: a meta-analysis with an emphasis on complications. Surgery. 2003;134(4):647–53; discussion 654–655.
32. Zheng X, Dou C, Yao Y, et al. A meta-analysis study of laparoscopic versus open splenectomy with or without esophagogastric devascularization in the management of liver cirrhosis and portal hypertension. J Laparoendosc Adv Surg Tech A. 2015;25(2):103–11.
33. Jiang GQ, Bai DS, Chen P, et al. Laparoscopic splenectomy and azygoportal disconnection: a systematic review. JSLS. 2015;19(4):pii: e2015.00091.
34. Al-raimi K, Zheng SS. Postoperative outcomes after open splenectomy versus laparoscopic splenectomy in cirrhotic patients: a meta-analysis. Hepatobiliary Pancreat Dis Int. 2016;15(1):14–20.
35. Yu H, Guo S, Wang L, et al. Laparoscopic splenectomy and esophagogastric devascularization for liver cirrhosis and portal hypertension is a safe, effective, and minimally invasive operation. J Laparoendosc Adv Surg Tech A. 2016;26(7):524–30.
36. Boyer TD, Habib S. Big spleens and hypersplenism: fix it or forget it? Liver Int. 2015;35(5):1492–8.
37. Townsend CM, Beauchamp RD, Evers BM, et al. Sabiston Textbook of Surgery: the biological basis of modern surgical practice. 20th ed. Amsterdam: Elsevier, Inc; 2017.
38. Wu MC, Wu ZD. Huang jiasi surgery. 7th ed. Beijing: People's Medical Publishing House; 2008.
39. Zhang QY. Qian Li abdominal surgery. 2nd ed. Beijing: People's Medical Publishing House; 2017.
40. Moris D, Dimitriou N, Griniatsos J. Laparoscopic splenectomy for benign hematological disorders in adults: a systematic review. In Vivo. 2017;31(3):291–302.
41. Weiss CA 3rd, Kavic SM, Adrales GL, et al. Laparoscopic splenectomy: what barriers remain? Surg Innov. 2005;12(1):23–9.
42. Dominguez EP, Choi YU, Scott BG, et al. Impact of morbid obesity on outcome of laparoscopic splenectomy. Surg Endosc. 2007;21(3):422–6.
43. Gernsheimer T, McCrae KR. Immune thrombocytopenic purpura in pregnancy. Curr Opin Hematol. 2007;14(5):574–80.
44. Yücel E, Kurt Y, Ozdemir Y, et al. Laparoscopic splenectomy for the treatment of wandering spleen in a pregnant woman: a case report. Surg Laparosc Endosc Percutan Tech. 2012;22(2):e102–4.
45. Majesky I, Daniel I, Stefanikova Z, et al. Laparoscopic splenectomy in pregnancy—from contraindication to golden standard. Bratisl Lek Listy. 2013;114(8):484–7.
46. Chen J, Ma R, Yang S, et al. Perioperative outcomes of laparoscopic versus open splenectomy for non-traumatic diseases: a meta-analysis. Chin Med J. 2014;127(13):2504–10.
47. Cheng J, Tao K, Yu P. Laparoscopic splenectomy is a better surgical approach for spleen-relevant disorders: a comprehensive meta-analysis based on 15-year literatures. Surg Endosc. 2016;30(10):4575–88.
48. Qian D, He Z, Hua J, et al. Hand-assisted versus conventional laparoscopic splenectomy: a systematic review and meta-analysis. ANZ J Surg. 2014;84(12):915–20.
49. Kusminsky RE, Boland JP, Tiley EH, et al. Hand-assisted laparoscopic splenectomy. Surg Laparosc Endosc. 1995;5(6):463–7.
50. Targarona EM, Lima MB, Balague C, et al. Single-port splenectomy: current update and controversies. J Minim Access Surg. 2011;7(1):61–4.
51. Fan Y, Wu SD, Kong J, et al. Feasibility and safety of single-incision laparoscopic splenectomy: a systematic review. J Surg Res. 2014;186(1):354–62.
52. Gkegkes ID, Mourtarakos S, Iavazzo C. Single-incision laparoscopic splenectomy. JSLS. 2014;18(3):e2014.00350.
53. Wu S, Lai H, Zhao J, et al. Systematic review and meta-analysis of single-incision versus conventional multiport laparoscopic splenectomy. J Minim Access Surg. 2018;14(1):1–8.
54. Barbaros U, Dinççağ A. Single incision laparoscopic splenectomy: the first two cases. J Gastrointest Surg. 2009;13(8):1520–3.
55. Bodner J, Kafka-Ritsch R, Lucciarini P, et al. A critical comparison of robotic versus conventional laparoscopic splenectomies. World J Surg. 2005;29(8):982–5; discussion 985–986
56. Gelmini R, Franzoni C, Spaziani A, et al. Laparoscopic splenectomy: conventional versus robotic approach—a comparative study. J Laparoendosc Adv Surg Tech A. 2011;21(5):393–8.
57. Giza DE, Tudor S, Purnichescu-Purtan RR, et al. Robotic splenectomy: what is the real benefit? World J Surg. 2014;38(12):3067–73.
58. Balaphas A, Buchs NC, Meyer J, et al. Partial splenectomy in the era of minimally invasive surgery: the current laparoscopic and robotic experiences. Surg Endosc. 2015;29(12):3618–27.

59. Christo MC. Partial regulated splenectomies. Preliminary note on the first 3 cases operated on [Article in Portuguese]. Hospital (Rio J). 1959;56:645–50.
60. Morgenstern L, Shapiro SJ. Partial splenectomy for nonparasitic splenic cysts. Am J Surg. 1980;139(2):278–81.
61. Poulin EC, Thibault C, DesCôteaux JG, et al. Partial laparoscopic splenectomy for trauma: technique and case report. Surg Laparosc Endosc. 1995;5(4):306–10.
62. Feng S, Qiu Y, Li X, et al. Laparoscopic versus open splenectomy in children: a systematic review and meta-analysis. Pediatr Surg Int. 2016;32(3):253–9.
63. Winslow ER, Brunt LM, Drebin JA, et al. Portal vein thrombosis after splenectomy. Am J Surg. 2002;184(6):631–5; discussion 635–636
64. Pietrabissa A, Moretto C, Antonelli G, et al. Thrombosis in the portal venous system after elective laparoscopic splenectomy. Surg Endosc. 2004;18(7):1140–3.
65. Harris W, Marcaccio M. Incidence of portal vein thrombosis after laparoscopic splenectomy. Can J Surg. 2005;48(5):352–4.
66. Romano F, Caprotti R, Scaini A, et al. Elective laparoscopic splenectomy and thrombosis of the splenoportal axis: a prospective study with ecocolordoppler ultrasound. Surg Laparosc Endosc Percutan Tech. 2006;16(1):4–7.
67. Ruiz-Tovar J, Pérez de Oteyza J, Blázquez Sánchez J, et al. Portal vein thrombosis after laparoscopic splenectomy in benign hematologic diseases. J Laparoendosc Adv Surg Tech A. 2007;17(4):448–54.
68. Svensson M, Wirén M, Kimby E, et al. Portal vein thrombosis is a common complication following splenectomy in patients with malignant haematological diseases. Eur J Haematol. 2006;77(3):203–9.
69. Ikeda M, Sekimoto M, Takiguchi S, et al. Total splenic vein thrombosis after laparoscopic splenectomy: a possible candidate for treatment. Am J Surg. 2007;193(1):21–5.
70. Danno K, Ikeda M, Sekimoto M, et al. Diameter of splenic vein is a risk factor for portal or splenic vein thrombosis after laparoscopic splenectomy. Surgery. 2009;145(5):457–64; discussion 465–466
71. Tran T, Demyttenaere SV, Polyhronopoulos G, et al. Recommended timing for surveillance ultrasonography to diagnose portal splenic vein thrombosis after laparoscopic splenectomy. Surg Endosc. 2010;24(7):1670–8.
72. Kawanaka H, Akahoshi T, Kinjo N, et al. Impact of antithrombin III concentrates on portal vein thrombosis after splenectomy in patients with liver cirrhosis and hypersplenism. Ann Surg. 2010;251(1):76–83.
73. Vecchio R, Cacciola E, Cacciola RR, et al. Portal vein thrombosis after laparoscopic and open splenectomy. J Laparoendosc Adv Surg Tech A. 2011;21(1):71–5.
74. Wang H, Kopac D, Brisebois R, et al. Randomized controlled trial to investigate the impact of anticoagulation on the incidence of splenic or portal vein thrombosis after laparoscopic splenectomy. Can J Surg. 2011;54(4):227–31.
75. Kakinoki K, Okano K, Suto H, et al. Hand-assisted laparoscopic splenectomy for thrombocytopenia in patients with cirrhosis. Surg Today. 2013;43(8): 883–8.
76. Alexakis N, Dardamanis D, Albanopoulos K, et al. Incidence, risk factors, and outcome of portal vein thrombosis after laparoscopic-assisted splenectomy in β-thalassemia patients: a prospective exploratory study. J Laparoendosc Adv Surg Tech A. 2013;23(2):123–8.
77. Cheng Z, Yu F, Tian J, et al. A comparative study of two anti-coagulation plans on the prevention of PVST after laparoscopic splenectomy and esophagogastric devascularization. J Thromb Thrombolysis. 2015;40(3):294–301.
78. Jiang GQ, Bai DS, Chen P, et al. Predictors of portal vein system thrombosis after laparoscopic splenectomy and azygoportal disconnection: a retrospective cohort study of 75 consecutive patients with 3-months follow-up. Int J Surg. 2016;30:143–9.
79. Manouchehri N, Kaneva P, Séguin C, et al. Screening for thrombophilia does not identify patients at risk of portal or splenic vein thrombosis following laparoscopic splenectomy. Surg Endosc. 2016;30(5): 2119–26.
80. de'Angelis N, Abdalla S, Lizzi V, et al. Incidence and predictors of portal and splenic vein thrombosis after pure laparoscopic splenectomy. Surgery. 2017;162(6):1219–30.
81. Qian YY, Li K. The early prevention and treatment of PVST after laparoscopic splenectomy: a prospective cohort study of 130 patients. Int J Surg. 2017;44:147–51.
82. Rottenstreich A, Kleinstern G, Spectre G, et al. Thromboembolic events following splenectomy: risk factors, prevention, management and outcomes. World J Surg. 2018;42(3):675–81.
83. Oomen MW, Bakx R, van Minden M, et al. Implementation of laparoscopic splenectomy in children and the incidence of portal vein thrombosis diagnosed by ultrasonography. J Pediatr Surg. 2013;48(11):2276–80.
84. Gelas T, Scalabre A, Hameury F, et al. Portal vein thrombosis after laparoscopic splenectomy during childhood. J Thromb Thrombolysis. 2014;38(2):218–22.
85. Kercher KW, Sing RF, Watson KW, et al. Transhepatic thrombolysis in acute portal vein thrombosis after laparoscopic splenectomy. Surg Laparosc Endosc Percutan Tech. 2002;12(2):131–6.

2 Anatomy and Physiology of the Spleen

Guoqing Ouyang, Wanlong Wu, and Bing Peng

2.1 Embryology and Clinical Anatomy of the Spleen

2.1.1 Embryology of the Spleen

The spleen is one of the asymmetric organs in the abdominal cavity and an important part of the lymphoid organs. From the view of embryology, however, it has the same origin as the digestive system. From the 5th week of an embryo, the spleen begins to form by gathering from mesoderm cells (mesenchymal cells) scattering in the dorsal mesentery of the stomach. The mesenchymal cells on the surface become multiple layers to form the spleen primordium. When the mesenchymal cell mass continues to divide and proliferate and gradually grows and expands, it protrudes into the abdominal cavity. The outer layer becomes the peritoneum, while the deep cells become splenic parenchyma, so that the splenic surface is covered with a layer of mesothelium. The spleen remains lobulated before birth; after birth, the lobule disappears, and only a small amount of groove named splenic notch is left on the upper edge of the spleen. When the dorsal margin of the stomach develops into greater curvature and the longitudinal axis of the stomach rotates from the front-back direction to the left-right direction, the dorsal mesentery of the stomach develops into gastric omental bursa and protrudes to the left, and the spleen is concomitantly pulled to the left lateral, namely, the left dorsal part of the stomach. The posterior lobe of the omental bursa fuses with the parietal layer and covers the left adrenal gland and the left kidney. The omentum between the stomach and the spleen evolves into the gastrosplenic ligament, while the omentum between the spleen and the parietal layer evolves into the lienorenal ligament.

2.1.2 Congenital Dysplasia of the Spleen

Understanding the congenital dysplasia of the spleen can be a reference for operation. There are several kinds of congenital anomalies of the spleen related to surgery.

2.1.2.1 Accessory Spleen

Accessory spleen is one or more spherical or hemispherical purple soft spleen nodules outside the normal spleen due to incomplete fusion of spleen primordia or ectopic spleen primordia. The accessory spleen is usually located in any position adjacent to the normal spleen, such as in the splenic hilum and gastrosplenic ligament (54%), splenic pedicle (25%), greater omentum (12%), tail of the pancreas (6%), splenocolic

G. Ouyang · W. Wu · B. Peng (✉)
West China Hospital, Sichuan University, Chengdu, China

B. Peng (ed.), *Laparoscopic Surgery of the Spleen*, https://doi.org/10.1007/978-981-16-1216-9_2

ligament (2%), mesentery (0.5%),or left ovary (0.5%) [1–3]. Some of the accessory spleens can be found ectopic in the liver, the pancreas, the left scrotum (the labia majora for the female), and the left testis, around the left fallopian tube, or even in the right chest. In rare cases, the accessory spleens are located in the spleen, i.e., hamartoma in the spleen. The incidence of the accessory spleen is from 15% to 35%. The younger has a higher incidence of the accessory spleen; however, the accessory spleen gets atrophy with age. If the accessory spleen is omitted during splenectomy, the residual accessory spleen may have compensatory growth and cause disease recurrence. Therefore, the suspicious accessory spleen should be explored and completely removed during a splenectomy for hypersplenism or hematological diseases.

The size of the accessory spleen varies from 0.2 to 10 cm. The number of the accessory spleen can be single or multiple, ranging from 1 to 6 or up to 10. Of the multiple accessory spleen cases, 85% occur in one site, and only 15% are found in two different sites [3, 4]. The occurrence of the accessory spleen in more than two sites has not been reported.

The accessory spleen may also undergo rupture, torsion, or infarction. Some reports have showed that the accessory spleen is suspected to be a mass above the kidney or a neoplasm within the greater curvature of the stomach; some other researches have demonstrated that torsion or spontaneous rupture of the accessory spleen may cause acute abdomen. If the accessory spleen is attached to the wall of gallbladder or near the hepatic hilum, it may cause compression symptoms and even obstructive jaundice. If the accessory spleen fuses with the intestinal wall, an intestinal obstruction or intussusception will occur. Rarely, the accessory spleen may pose urinary tract obstruction.

2.1.2.2 Asplenia and Polysplenia

Asplenia and polysplenia are often associated with partial situs inversus viscerum, which is a rare dysplasia and is the result of the spleen primordium not forming (without spleen) or not fusing (multiple spleen) before the 6th week of an embryo. In children, asplenia may be asymptomatic, but the immune function is weak, thus easily forming fulminant infection. In adults, asplenia is rare and often accidentally found during other intraperitoneal operations.

Polysplenia is a single leafy spleen or a spleen composed of 2–9 independent but approximately equal-sized splenic masses, often accompanied by the development of asymmetric organs such as the heart, the lung, the bronchus, the liver, the bile duct, the stomach, the pancreas, and the intestine. More than 3/4 of the patients with polysplenia die before the age of 5, and 50% of them survive for less than 4 months [2], so it is rare in adults.

Polysplenia itself does not produce clinical symptoms, and its clinical importance only presents when the concurrent deformity of the heart, the lung, or the gastrointestinal tract needs a surgical operation. Polysplenia should be differentiated with accessory spleen and the splenic autotransplantation secondary to splenic rupture or splenectomy. The fragments of a ruptured spleen may scatter on the surface of abdominal organs, the greater omentum, or peritoneum and sometimes cover the full abdominal cavity. With the number of tens to hundreds, the autotransplantation splenic tissue can survive, grow, and proliferate into multiple small nodules, showing the spleen tissue structure and irregular shape without the splenic hilum. Splenectomy and autologous spleen transplantation is mainly performed on condition that a traumatic splenic rupture endangers the patient's life. In order to maintain the spleen function and avoid the overwhelming post-splenectomy infection (OPSI) and immunologic dysfunction after surgery, the autologous splenic tissue is intentionally selected and cut into little pieces and then placed between the anterior and posterior layer of the greater omentum during the splenectomy.

2.1.2.3 Wandering Spleen

Wandering spleen or ectopic spleen, mainly happening in multipara, is defined as the spleen which leaves away from the original normal anatomical position to other parts of the abdominal cavity or the pelvis. It is related to the development defect of the dorsal mesentery of the stomach, as well as multiple pregnancies, emaciation, and weakness of the abdominal muscles. Splenic ligament relaxation caused by splenic disease (such as splenomegaly) or trauma or splenic ligament deficiency can also generate wandering spleen. This disease is more common in women especially the multipara than men. The most common wandering positions of the spleen are left upper middle abdomen, right middle abdomen, left lower abdomen, and pelvis. Sometimes a wandering spleen can go even down to the right lower abdomen and enter the left scrotum along the left groin or herniate into the chest through the diaphragm hiatus. If the wandering spleen is twisted, it may induce acute abdomen. The sign of a wandering spleen is an asymptomatic mass in the abdominal cavity, which can move with the change of body position during physical examination and can be easily pushed back to the left upper quadrant. The wandering spleen should be differentiated with gynecological tumor, renal tumor, mesenteric tumor, and intestinal neoplasm.

2.1.2.4 Fusion of the Spleen Tissues with Organs

There is splenogonadal fusion, spleen liver fusion, spleen kidney fusion, and spleen peritoneum fusion. Splenogonadal fusion (SGF) is due to the abnormal adhesion of the two primordial urogenital ridges, which are close to the gonad during the process of the spleen evolution and the dorsal mesentery rotating to the left. The fusion of the spleen and gonad almost occurs on the left side of the male. SGF can be categorized into two types: ① Connected type, the normal spleen connects to the left testis or scrotum with a continuous spleen tissue or connective tissue cord between the gonad and the normal spleen; and ② unconnected type, spleen tissue fuses with the gonad, but there is no intermediate connecting cord between the gonad and the normal spleen organ. The connecting cord between the spleen and the gonad can induce mechanical intestinal obstruction, so the connecting cord must be cut off through surgery [3–5]. Any mass in the scrotum, especially on the left side, should be suspected as SGF.

2.1.3 Clinical Anatomy of the Spleen

2.1.3.1 Shape, Position, and Adjacency of the Spleen

The spleen, like a broad bean, is the largest lymphoid organ of human body. The red pulp and white pulp account for 75% and 20%, respectively. The spleen is dark red, soft, and fragile. Generally, the adult spleen is about 12 cm in length, 7 cm in width, 3–4 cm in thickness, and 110–200 g in weight [3]. The spleen is located in the posterolateral of the left costal region between the stomach and the diaphragm and cannot be touched under the costal margin in normal physical examination. Covered by the left costal arch from the front, the spleen is corresponding to the 9th to the 11th ribs, and the long axis of it is consistent with the 10th rib [1]. The spleen is about 2.5 cm lower in upright position than in supine position. The posterior end of the spleen is parallel to the ninth lumbar spine and about 4–5 cm away from the posterior midline; the anterior end is parallel to the first lumbar spine and is not beyond the axillary midline. The lower pole of the spleen is located at the 11th rib of the left anterior axillary line. Of the diaphragmatic surface of the spleen, the upper 1/3 is covered by the lower edge of the left lung, the middle 1/3 is covered by the left costophrenic recess, and the lower 1/3 is covered by the lower boundary of the pleura and the starting point of the costophrenic part [3–9].

The spleen has two surfaces (diaphragmatic surface and visceral surface), two edges (anterior edge and posterior edge), and two poles (upper pole and lower pole). The diaphragmatic surface is convex and close to the diaphragm. A strike on the left lower part of the chest or the left upper quadrant may cause splenic rupture. The front visceral surface (stomach surface) contacts with the fundus of the stomach, and the back visceral surface (kidney surface) contacts with the left kidney and the front of the left adrenal gland. Splenic hilum is the site where the blood vessels, nervous bunches, and lymphatic vessels (the blood vessels, nervous bunches, and lymphatic vessels are collectively called as splenic

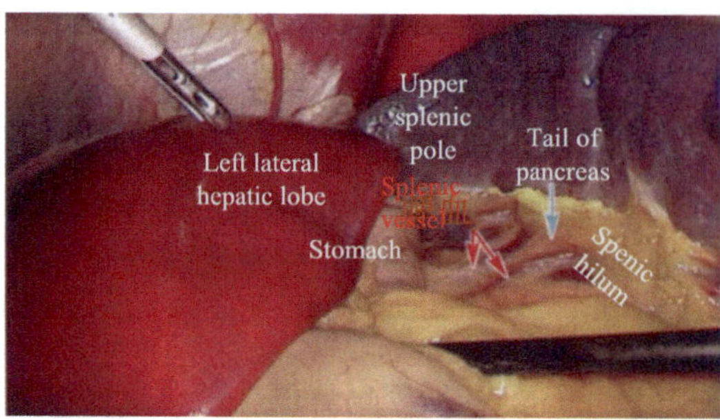

Fig. 2.1 Anatomy of the splenic hilum

pedicle) of the spleen enter and exit the spleen (Fig. 2.1). The anterior edge of the spleen is thin and sharp, obliquely inserting upward into the space between the fundus of the stomach and the diaphragm and extending downward between the splenic flexure of the transverse colon and the diaphragm. When the left lateral hepatic lobe becomes hypertrophied, part of the anterior edge of the spleen can be covered by the hypertrophic liver lobe. Sometimes it is necessary to dissect the left lateral hepatic lobe and reverse it to the right to acquire full exposure of the upper pole of the spleen. The posterior edge of the spleen is blunt and obliquely downward. The upper pole of the spleen is blunt and round, and the lower pole is slightly sharp.

The splenic hilum is adjacent to the tail of the pancreas. In 50% cases, the tail of the pancreas is about 1 cm away from the splenic hilum; in about 1/3 cases, the tail of the pancreas is in direct contact with the splenic hilum. In the remaining cases, 49.5% are close to the center of the splenic hilum, 42.25% close to the lower pole of the spleen, and 8.25% close to the upper pole of the spleen [1, 6]. Attention should be paid to prevent the tail of the pancreas from being damaged by mistake during splenectomy.

2.1.3.2 Ligaments of the Spleen

The spleen is an intraperitoneal organ. Except for the splenic hilum, most of the splenic surface is covered by peritoneum. The ligaments of the spleen are formed by retroperitoneal fold, and according to the relationship with adjacent organs, they can be respectively called as the gastrosplenic ligament, the lienorenal ligament (also written as the splenorenal ligament), the splenophrenic ligament, the splenocolic ligament, the anterior spleen plica, the pancreaticosplenic ligament, the phrenicocolic ligament, and the pancreaticocolic ligament. The length, width, and mutual contact of the ligaments may vary. The extent of activity of the spleen depends on the relaxation of the ligaments of the spleen and the length of the splenic vessels.

Gastrosplenic Ligament

The gastrosplenic ligament originates from the dorsal mesentery of the stomach in the embryonic period, forming a triangle between the stomach and the spleen and extending from the left side of the greater curvature of the stomach to the splenic hilum. The two layers of peritoneum are separated by splenic hilum. The anterior layer wraps the whole spleen to form the serosal layer of the spleen and turns into the posterior layer of the lienorenal ligament at the lower margin of the splenic hilum. On the other hand, the posterior layer of the gastrosplenic ligament covers the splenic artery inward at the splenic hilum and transits into the peritoneum of the posterior wall of the omental bursa and the anterior layer of the lienorenal ligament (Fig. 2.2). Inside the gastrosplenic ligament, there are short gastric vessels in the upper part and left gastroepiploic vessels in the lower part. During the separation of the gastrosplenic ligament, the above vessels should be carefully ligated to avoid bleeding and injury to the gastric wall.

Lienorenal Ligament

The lienorenal ligament consists of two layers, one is the anterior layer, and the other is the posterior

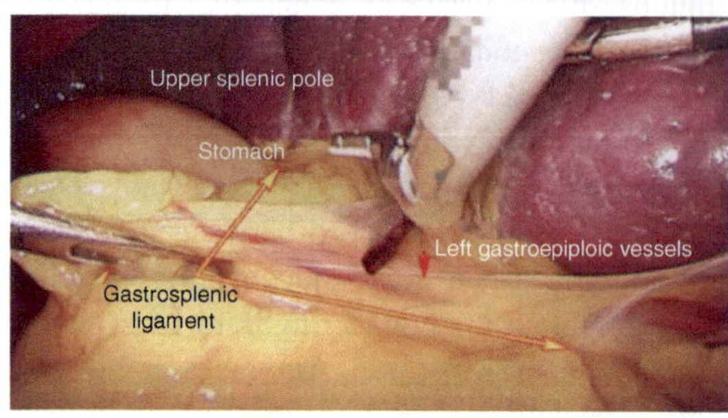

Fig. 2.2 Gastrosplenic ligament

layer. The anterior layer originates from the posterior layer of the gastrosplenic ligament which is described in detail in the above paragraph; the posterior layer is the peritoneum (the anterior layer of the gastrosplenic ligament) that encloses the spleen, which turns to form the ligament at the posterior lower edge of the splenic hilum. There are splenic arteries and veins inside the lienorenal ligament. Sometimes the tail of the pancreas can extend into the lienorenal ligament and reach the splenic hilum (Figs. 2.3 and 2.4). The anterior layer of the lienorenal ligament extends to the right and covers the front of the pancreas. If the tail of the pancreas does not directly contact the spleen, the anterior layer is called the pancreaticosplenic ligament. There are branches of the pancreatic tail artery in the pancreaticosplenic ligament. During the operation, the branches of the pancreatic tail artery should be carefully separated and ligated to avoid damage to the tail of the pancreas. The lienorenal ligament is short; when splenectomy is performed, the posterior layer of the lienorenal ligament should be cut open first to free the spleen and overturn it.

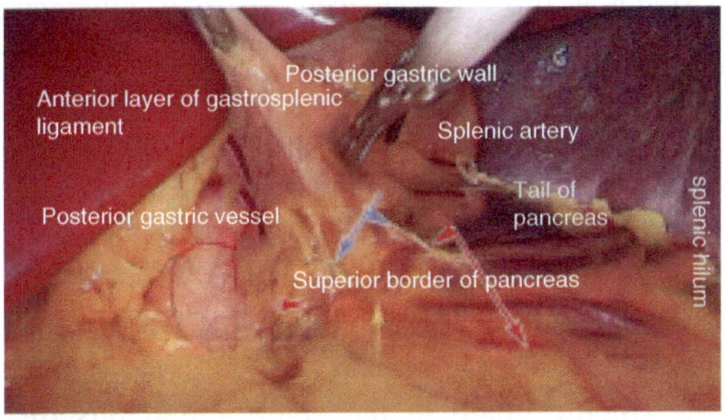

Fig. 2.3 Anterior layer of lienorenal ligament

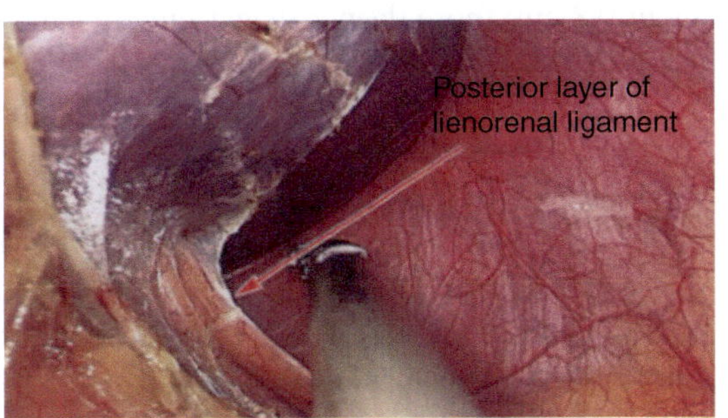

Fig. 2.4 Posterior layer of lienorenal ligament

Splenophrenic Ligament

The splenophrenic ligament is the peritoneal plica extending from the lienorenal ligament to the diaphragm and is located between the cardia and the upper pole of the spleen (Fig. 2.5). The splenophrenic ligament contains smooth muscle fibers and sometimes includes the cardia branch and esophageal branch of the inferior phrenic artery. This ligament is short, and in order to free the upper pole of the spleen, it must be cut off. The ligation after cutoff should be firm to avoid hemorrhaging.

Splenocolic Ligament

The splenocolic ligament is the part of the lower left part of the gastrosplenic ligament that extends downward to the greater omentum and is located between the lower pole of the spleen and the splenic flexure of the transverse colon (Fig. 2.6). Sometimes the blood vessels of the lower pole of the spleen or the left gastroepiploic artery cling to the ligament. When cutting off the ligament, pay attention not to hurt the blood vessels and the transverse colon.

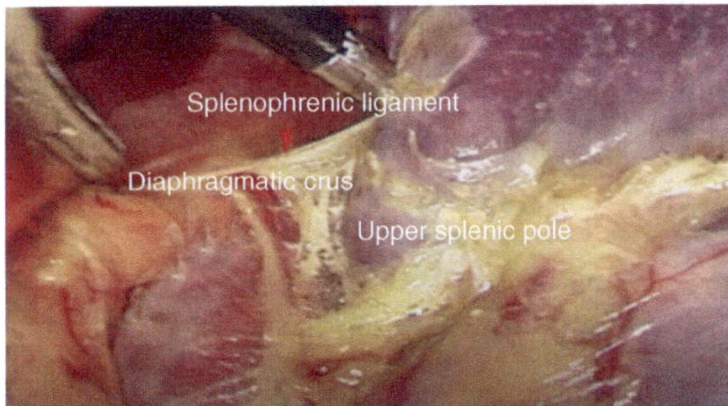

Fig. 2.5 Splenophrenic ligament

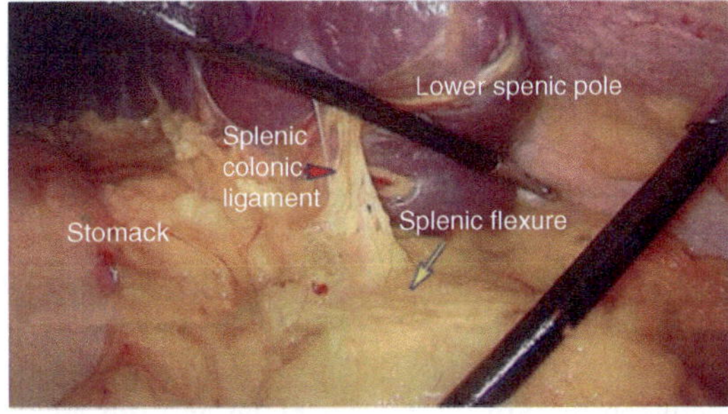

Fig. 2.6 Splenocolic ligament

Anterior Spleen Plica

The anterior spleen plica is the peritoneal plica in front of the gastrosplenic ligament. A long splenic pedicle often has the anterior splenic plica. There is a branch of the left gastroepiploic artery in it, which is easy to cause bleeding due to over traction.

Phrenicocolic Ligament

The phrenicocolic ligament is a peritoneal fold extending between the costal part of the diaphragm and the splenic flexure of the transverse colon. This ligament supports the spleen from beneath it and plays a certain role in maintaining the normal position of the spleen. As the spleen continues to grow and develop, the ligament is gradually pouching and seems like a hammock. As it extends between the splenic flexure and phren, it can block the hematocelia flow freely through the upper and lower region of the colon. If the phrenicocolic ligament is too short, the lower pole of the spleen will be closely adjoined to the splenic flexure and may be damaged during splenectomy.

Pancreaticocolic Ligament

The pancreaticocolic ligament is a plica extending from the upper part of the mesocolon and just between the pancreas and the transverse colon.

2.1.3.3 Lobes and Segments of the Spleen

According to the distribution of the splenic lobar arteries and the splenic segmental arteries in the corresponding areas of the spleen, the spleen is divided into the upper lobe and lower lobe or the upper lobe, middle lobe, and lower lobe. If the spleen is of four segments, it is also divided into upper, upper middle, lower middle, and lower segments (see Sect. 2.2 for details).

2.1.3.4 Sectional Anatomy of the Spleen

Marked by ribs and intercostals, the spleen can reach as high as the 8th costal plane and as low as the 12th costal plane. Usually, the spleen appears between the 8th intercostal plane and 9th costal plane and disappears at the 11th costal plane. Marked by the vertebral body, the spleen can appear as high as the T_{10} level or as low as the L_2 to L_3 level. It usually appears between the T_{10} to T_{11} intervertebral disc and the T_{11} level and disappears at the L_1 to L_2 level.

2.1.3.5 Splenic Notch

The appearance of splenic notch is closely related to the development of the spleen. At the 3rd month of an embryo, the notches have already formed, and from then on, most of the notches have gradually disappeared. The splenic notch can be found in the anterior edge, posterior edge, as well as diaphragmatic surface. The occurrence rate of notches in the anterior edge is as high as 84%, and the number of such notches varies from 1 to 5 (3 in most cases), usually seen in the lower middle 1/3 of the anterior edge; it is a sign to distinguish whether the left upper abdominal mass is an enlarged spleen. The occurrence rate of notches in the posterior edge is 21.1–59.2%, and the number of such notches is usually 1 (3 in some cases), usually seen in the upper 1/3 of the posterior edge. If the posterior splenic notch extends to the visceral surface, it is usually connected with the extension line of the relative anterior splenic notch to form a lobar boundary. The occurrence rate of notches in the diaphragmatic surface is about 10%, and the number of such notches is usually 1, usually seen in the upper 1/3 of the diaphragmatic surface. Occasionally, the splenic notch in the diaphragmatic surface goes deep into the splenic parenchyma and connects the splenic notch in the anterior and posterior edge to form two splenic lobes [1].

The depth of the shallow splenic notch is about 0.8 cm; those deeper than 1 cm are called deep splenic notch. The deep splenic notch is mainly located between the two lobes, and the coincidence rate of deep splenic notch with interlobar and intersegmental fissures is 94.92%. In 87% of the cases, splenic notch passes through less vascular area, and the extension line of the splenic notch can be used as a reference for the demarcation line in lobectomy or segmentectomy of the spleen [1].

2.2 Blood Supply, Lymphatic Circulation, and Innervation of the Spleen

2.2.1 Blood Vessels of the Spleen

The splenic artery and the splenic vein are both single. The normal splenic artery originates from the celiac trunk, and the splenic vein converges into the portal vein.

2.2.1.1 Splenic Artery

The splenic artery originates from the celiac trunk (98.98% in Chinese people) and very few from the abdominal aorta (0.28%) or the superior mesenteric artery (0.65%). The average length of the splenic artery in Chinese is 12.1 cm (7.1–39.2 cm), and 11–16 cm accounts for 62% [3]. The diameter of the initial part of the splenic artery is 4–20 mm, with an average of (8.07 ± 2.19) mm. The diameter of the terminal part is 3.5–14.5 mm, with an average of (6.01 ± 1.87) mm [1].

Course of the Splenic Artery

Most of the trunks of the splenic arteries curve in varying degrees. The splenic arteries in infants do not curve, but gradually curve with age. After the splenic artery arising from the celiac trunk, it goes down to the superior margin of the pancreas. Then along the superior posterior margin and above the splenic vein, 60% of the splenic artery goes to left until entering the splenic hilum, a part of the splenic artery goes through the anterior pancreas (30%) or the posterior pancreas (8%), and a few are embedded in the pancreatic parenchyma [1]. The trunk of the splenic artery can be divided into four segments according to its course:

1. Upper segment of the pancreas: This segment is from the celiac trunk to the pancreas. It's very short and about 1–3 cm long [3, 7]. It usually curves anticlockwise with concave surface upward, then passes through the front of the abdominal aorta, and continues to the upper edge of the dorsal side of the pancreas to become the pancreatic segment. In this segment, the left inferior phrenic artery, the dorsal pancreatic artery, the superior polar splenic artery, the posterior gastric artery, the accessory hepatic artery, or the inferior mesenteric artery can be produced.
2. Pancreatic segment: This is the longest segment of the splenic artery. In this segment, the splenic artery runs to the left across the posterior superior margin of the pancreas, presenting one or more loops in adults. This segment can give out the great pancreatic artery, the posterior gastric artery, the short gastric artery, or the left gastric artery.
3. Anterior segment of the pancreas: It is a short segment of the splenic artery that moves obliquely to the left in front of the tail of the pancreas. If the splenic artery is divided into terminal branches here, it is categorized as dispersive type, and 70% of the cases are of this type [1, 3]. The characteristics of this segment lie in that the trunk of the splenic artery is relatively short and it is difficult to ligate during operation; the length of the terminal arteries' trunk is long, the branches of the terminal arteries are also long, and the number of the branches is large; accordingly, the sites of the branches entering the spleen are scattered. The anterior segment of the pancreas can generate the left gastroepiploic artery, the superior polar splenic artery, the short gastric artery, and the pancreatic tail artery.
4. Segment before the splenic hilum: The segment is between the tail of the pancreas and the splenic hilum. If the splenic artery is divided into terminal branches here, then it is categorized as compact type, and 30% of the cases are of this type [1, 3]. For this type, the splenic artery trunk is relatively long, the terminal artery and its branches are relatively short, and the number of branches is small. The spleen of this type often has no notches or superior and inferior polar splenic arteries.

The course of the splenic artery is closely related to the pancreas. The distance between the proximal 1/4 of the splenic artery and the pancreas and the splenic vein is relatively long, while the distance between the distal 3/4 of the splenic artery is relatively short, but the variation is large. According to the variation, it is often divided into four types. Type I: This type accounts for 47% of the cases; the splenic artery runs along the superior margin of the pancreas to the splenic hilum after it originates from the celiac trunk. Type II: This type accounts for 14% of the cases; the middle 2/4 of the splenic artery is located behind or in the pancreas. Type III: This type accounts for 6%; the distal 2/4 of the splenic artery is located behind or in the pancreas. Type IV: This type accounts for 33%; the distal 3/4 of the splenic artery is located behind or in the pancreas [1].

Branches of the Splenic Artery

There may be multiple branches in the course of the splenic artery, including the dorsal pancreatic artery, the great pancreatic artery, the pancreatic tail artery, the pancreatic branches, the superior polar splenic artery, the inferior polar splenic artery, the short gastric artery, the posterior gastric artery, and the left gastroepiploic artery.

With the wide development of vascular casting technology and the application of angiography technology, there are many studies on the branches and distribution of blood vessels in the spleen in recent years. These studies also promote the development of spleen preservation technology.

1. Splenic lobar artery and splenic segmental artery: According to the distribution of the supply area of the terminal branches of the splenic artery in the spleen, the spleen is divided into several splenic lobes. Before entering the splenic hilum, most of the splenic arteries are divided into two terminal branches, and only a few are divided into three terminal branches. These terminal branches are called splenic lobar arteries (class I branches). According to these lobar arteries, the spleen is divided into upper lobe and lower lobe or upper lobe, middle lobe, and lower lobe. The number of splenic lobar arteries can vary, so it can be divided into one-branch type, two-branch type, or three-branch type. One-branch type is rare and accounts for 3–5.17% of the cases. Two-branch type is more common and accounts for 76–98% of the cases. Three-branch type is rare and accounts for 2–23.18% of the cases. Multi-branch type is very rare [3–5, 8, 9]. Then, according to the distribution of the branches of the splenic lobar artery (class I branches) in the spleen, the spleen is further divided into splenic segments. The arteries supplying the corresponding splenic segments are called splenic segmental arteries (class II branches). There are usually 1–3 splenic segmental arteries in each splenic lobe, and there are (6 ± 0.1516) splenic segmental arteries in each spleen on average [1]. The most common segmental arteries are four-segment arteries; that is, the superior lobar splenic artery is divided into the upper and upper middle splenic segmental arteries, and the inferior lobar splenic artery is divided into the lower and lower middle splenic segmental arteries. Each splenic segment has a segmental artery and a segmental vein, which, together with the splenic tissue of the corresponding region, constitute a relatively independent morphological unit. The adjacent splenic segments are "relatively avascular plane," which is the anatomical basis of spleen preservation surgery (lobectomy or segmentectomy). The embolization of a certain splenic segmental artery can cause the infarction of the splenic segment in its blood supply range.
2. Splenic polar artery: The splenic polar artery is the artery that directly enters the upper and lower poles of the spleen without passing through the splenic hilum. The occurrence rate of the superior splenic polar artery is 14–62%, its length is about 2.7–15.4 cm, and its diameter is about 1.56 mm. Most of the superior polar arteries originate from the trunk of the splenic artery, and a few originate from the superior splenic lobar artery. If they originate from the celiac trunk (2%), they are called the dual splenic artery or the second splenic artery. Some may originate from the upper splenic segmental artery. The occurrence rate of the inferior splenic polar artery is

22–82%, its length is 2.4–9.7 cm, and its diameter is about 1.52 mm. The inferior splenic polar artery usually originates from the left gastroepiploic artery, followed by the inferior splenic lobar artery or the trunk of the splenic artery [2].

The splenic polar artery has important clinical significance because of the following reasons. First, when the splenic polar artery alone supplies the upper or lower part of the spleen, the polar artery must be properly protected to avoid the failure of the spleen preservation operation. Second, when the vasculature near the splenic hilum is ligated, it is easy to tear the polar artery and cause bleeding. Third, when the splenectomy is performed, surgeons may ignore the existence of the polar artery and unintentionally damage it, thus causing serious bleeding during the operation.

The branches of the splenic artery, such as the short gastric artery, the left gastroepiploic artery, and the pancreatic tail artery, sometimes do not originate from the trunk of the splenic artery, but from a certain splenic branch or polar artery. During splenectomy, the origin of above vessels should be identified, and the stump of these vessels should be properly ligated to avoid bleeding.

2.2.1.2 Splenic Vein

The splenic segmental veins accompany with the splenic segmental arteries, and finally the splenic segmental veins form into 2–3 lobar veins (splenic branches) in the spleen. The lobar veins go out of the splenic hilum and merge into the splenic vein in the splenorenal ligament. The average length between the confluence point and the midpoint of the splenic hilum is 3.4 cm [3, 6, 8]. The splenic vein is larger and straighter than the splenic artery; and it runs beneath the splenic artery to the right and reaches the back of the pancreatic neck. Then the splenic vein converges with the superior mesenteric vein at nearly a right angle to form the portal vein. Along the course, the splenic vein receives blood flux from the splenic polar vein, the branches of pancreatic vein, the short gastric vein, the posterior gastric vein, the left gastroepiploic vein, and the inferior mesenteric vein. Sometimes the left gastric vein can flow into the spleen vein before the splenic vein converging to the superior mesenteric vein. The length of the trunk of the splenic vein is 4.3–9.8 cm, and the average length is 8.1 cm. The diameter of the trunk of the splenic vein is 0.5–1 cm, and the average diameter is 0.7 cm [1].

The splenic vein goes with the splenic artery, both are closely related, and there are three types of anatomical relationship between them:

1. The splenic vein runs completely in the back of the splenic artery and is mostly located in the transverse sulcus of the pancreas or sometimes in the pancreatic parenchyma. This type accounts for 54% of the cases.
2. The splenic vein runs around the splenic artery. Part of the splenic vein runs in front of the artery and part of splenic vein runs behind the splenic artery. This type accounts for 44% of the cases.
3. The splenic vein runs completely in front of the splenic artery. This type accounts for 2% of the cases [1].

2.2.1.3 Double Circulation Pathway of the Spleen

It has been proved that in addition to the blood circulation of the splenic arteriovenous trunk system, the blood circulation pathway formed by the short gastric artery and vein, the left gastroepiploic artery and vein, the posterior gastric artery and vein, and the right gastroepiploic artery and vein through the gastroepiploic vascular arch is the most important side circulation of the spleen. In order to ensure the blood perfusion of the spleen, we should pay special attention to protect the short gastric vessels and the left gastroepiploic vessels in the gastrosplenic ligament when performing spleen preserved distal pancreatectomy for distal pancreatic cancer.

2.2.1.4 Division of the Spleen

According to the branching system of the blood vessels in the spleen, the thickness, as well as the width of the spleen, Dixon has divided the spleen from the visceral surface to the diaphragmatic surface into three divisions:

1. Splenic hilum division: the place where the spleen lobar, the segmental, and most of the subsegmental vessels pass through
2. Middle division: the place where is located a few of the subsegmental vessels, the trabecular vessels, the central arteries, and the small veins
3. Peripheral division: the place where the arteriae penicilli (medullary arteries, sheath arteries, and arterial capillaries), the sheath vein, and the blood sinuses are located [1, 6]

Based on the divisions and their compositional blood vessels, the bleeding from the superficial laceration no more than 1 cm in the peripheral division can be stopped with fine fibrous collagen, PW spray glue, or fibrin glue. The blood in the middle division can be coagulated with electrocoagulation, laser, or silver clip. If necessary, it is advisable to ligate the bleeding vessels. However, the bleeding in the splenic hilum division must be stopped by ligating. The divisions of the spleen therefore have certain clinical value and can provide anatomic basis for splenic bioadhesion, splenic repairment, or various irregular splenectomy.

2.2.2 Lymphatic Circulation of the Spleen

There is no lymphatic duct in the splenic parenchyma and medulla. The capsule and trabecular lymphatics of the spleen are integrated with the lymphatics accompanying the splenic artery and vein and then flow into the lymph nodes located at the splenic hilum and the superior margin of the pancreas. After that, the lymph flows into the lymph nodes along the splenic artery and finally into the lymph nodes around the celiac trunk.

2.2.3 Innervation of the Spleen

The innervation of the spleen is the sympathetic innervation, and the sympathetic nerve comes from the inner and anterior part of the celiac plexus. The nerve fiber bundle separated from the celiac plexus surrounds the splenic artery and is called the splenic plexus. It branches into the spleen along with the splenic artery and is distributed in the splenic capsule, trabecula, and blood vessels. It also branches along with the blood vessels and reaches the smooth muscle of the central artery and the medullary artery. When stimulated, these branches induce the contraction of the smooth muscle. The right vagus nerve or the posterior trunk of the vagus nerve also enters the spleen and is distributed in the smooth muscle of the branches of the splenic artery. The terminal branch of the left phrenic nerve (sensory fiber) reaches the splenophrenic ligament, so the spleen lesion or hemorrhage from spleen rupture can stimulate the phrenic nerve and cause the left shoulder referred pain (the Kehr's sign).

2.3 Physiology of the Spleen

The spleen is a highly vascularized organ which has the function of storing and filtering blood, and it can store about 20% of the whole blood volume [1]. Four- to five percent of the per minute cardiac output passes through the spleen and may amount to 200–300 mL/100 g of the spleen tissue. In adults, the daily blood volume flowing through the spleen can reach as large as 250 L; 10% of the blood flow directly enters the collateral veins after passing through the splenic cord, and 90% of the blood flow enters the red pulp, then slowly flowing back into the splenic vein [2]. The size of the spleen is discrepant. The blood storage capacity varies from dozens of ml to thousands of ml [1], with an average of 150–200 mL [2]. Under pathological condition, such as the enlarged spleen secondary to portal hypertension, the amount of stored blood volume can be increased by as much as tenfold [2], which can partially relieve the pressure of the blood vessels around the cardia and reduce the possibility of upper gastrointestinal hemorrhage. The filtration of red blood cells by the spleen is selective. Old or broken red blood cells and foreign particles are phagocytized and removed by phagocytes in the splenic sinuses and splenic cords.

The spleen is also an important hematopoietic and blood cells destroying organ. In fetal period, especially in the 2nd to 5th month, the spleen is one of the organs of extramedullary hematopoiesis; after the 5th month, the function of hematopoiesis is weakened [1]. After hematopoiesis, hematopoietic stem cells turn into a dormant state. After birth, only lymphocytes and monocytes are produced in the spleen. However, under stress or pathological conditions, such as massive blood loss, hemolysis, severe thalassemia, or myelofibrosis, the spleen can recover its hematopoietic function again. The spleen can also destroy blood cells, which is the main place to remove aging and broken red blood cells. When the spleen is enlarged, the blood flowing through the spleen becomes slower, extending from the normal 5 min to 1 h [2]. In addition, the blood cells destroying function of the spleen is strengthened, and even normal red blood cells will be destroyed. In hypersplenism, reticuloendothelial cells are hyperactive, the effect of destroying blood cells is also intensified, and even the leukocytes and platelets are destroyed. After splenectomy, the circulating leukocytes and platelets will rise.

The reticuloendothelial system of the spleen is well developed and has important immune function. The spleen can secrete some bioactive factors, such as tuftsin, opsonin, properdin, fibronectin, complement, cyclic adenosine monophosphate (cAMP), cyclic guanosine monophosphate (cGMP), immune ribonucleic acid (IRNA), as well as endogenous cytotoxic factors. These bioactive factors may promote the phagocytosis of foreign bodies and antigen-presenting function of monocytes, macrophages, and dendritic cells. Moreover, the spleen is the largest lymphoid organ in the human body and is the only lymphoid organ in the blood channel, so that it can produce a large number of T-lymphocytes and B-lymphocytes. T cells play a specific cellular immune function, while B cells play a specific humoral immune function [1, 2].

With the understanding of the overwhelming postsplenectomy infection (OPSI) after splenectomy, the important role of spleen in anti-infection has been clarified and thus promotes the widespread acceptance of the concept of "spleen preservation." Total splenectomy is not recommended for children under 4 years old. It has long been reported that in the early stage of gastric cancer, the spleen can inhibit the progression of tumor; however, in the late stage of gastric cancer, the spleen is a factor promoting the progression of tumor [10]. Therefore, the spleen plays a "bidirectional" and "phasic" role in tumor immunity, but its specific mechanism is still under investigation. Moreover, the spleen also has certain endocrine function which is an important part of the neuroendocrine-immune regulatory pathway of the body, and it can maintain the homeostasis. In addition, the spleen is also associated with the liver, the pancreas, the lung, the intestine, other lymphoid organs, and the endocrine organs. Their functional mechanism has not yet been fully studied and needs further research [1].

2.4 Imaging Anatomy of the Spleen

2.4.1 Ultrasonography Anatomy of the Spleen

Supine position or right 45°position is the most common used position in ultrasonography. ① Left intercostal oblique section check: Continuous scan of the axillary midline among the 9th to 11th intercostal can show the largest longitudinal section through the splenic hilum. The splenic hilum vessels and their branches and the tail of the pancreas can also be shown in this section. When the left hepatic lobe is enlarged, the hepatic lobe with slightly discrepant echo from the splenic parenchyma can be seen between the spleen and the diaphragm, which is easy to be mistaken for the abnormal or enlarged spleen echo. ② Longitudinal scan of the left hypochondrial region check: The upper pole of the spleen, the upper pole of the kidney, and the splenic hilum can be shown through this check. This section must be scanned when differentiating masses of the spleen with the masses of the kidney and discovering splenorenal shunt.

Under ultrasonography, the normal spleen presents crescent shape, clear outline, smooth surface, and medium parenchyma echo. The echo of the spleen is slightly lower than that of the hepatic tissue (Fig. 2.7); the upper part of the spleen is close to the diaphragm and is easily obscured by the gas in the lung tissue; the diameter of the vein in the splenic hilum section is less than 0.8 cm and has 2–6 branches; and the diameter of the splenic artery in the splenic hilum section is 0.3–0.4 cm, and the splenic artery has 2–3 branches. Color Doppler ultrasound can show the blood flow of the splenic hilum (Fig. 2.8). The thickness of the spleen measured by ultrasonography is the vertical distance from the splenic hilum to the tangent line of the opposite edge, and the normal reference value of thickness ranges from 3 to 4 cm; the long axis is the distance from the highest point of the upper pole of the spleen to the lowest point of the lower pole of the spleen; the width of the spleen is the maximum distance perpendicular to the long axis. If the maximum long axis is more than 11 cm in ultrasonographic images, it can be judged as splenomegaly. The echo intensity of the accessory spleen is the same as that of the normal spleen, shown as a round or oval homogeneous echo.

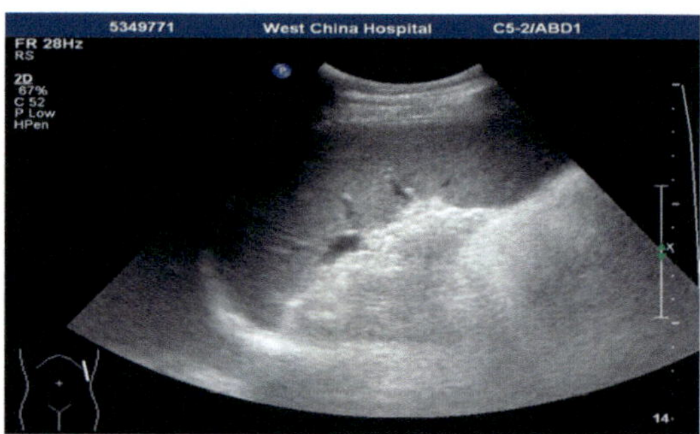

Fig. 2.7 Ultrasonographic image of the normal spleen

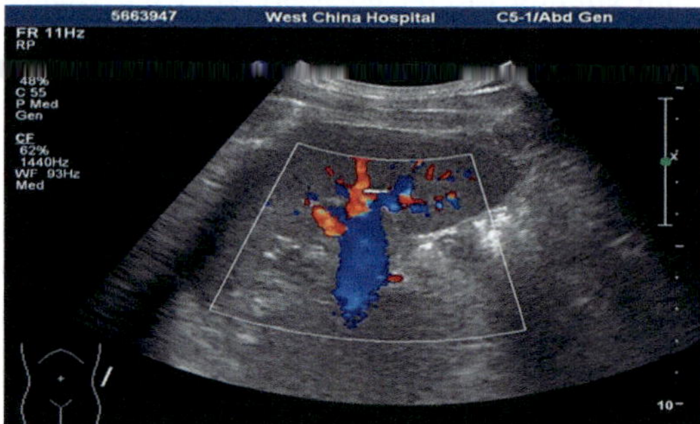

Fig. 2.8 Ultrasonographic image of the normal splenic hilum blood flow

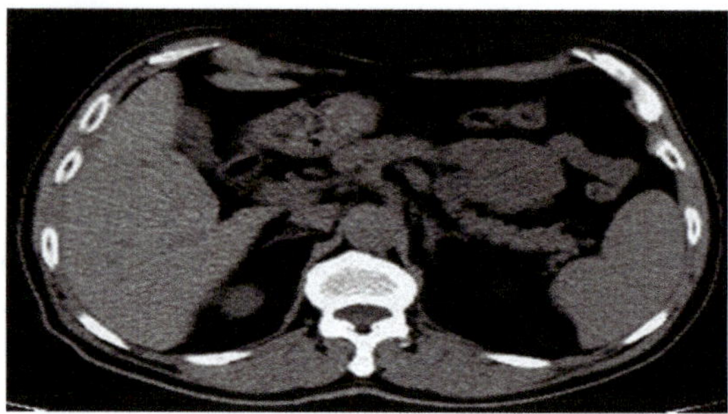

Fig. 2.9 CT image of the normal spleen (through splenic the hilum section)

2.4.2 CT Anatomy of the Spleen

The shape of the spleen on CT cross section varies from sections: the upper part and the lower part of the spleen are crescent shaped; the middle part (splenic hilum) is semi-circular or oval with concave inner edge. The CT value of the spleen is (45 ± 5) Hu, equal to or less than that of the liver. On CT cross section, a rib as well as an intercostal space is called one rib unit. The long axis of the spleen is equal to five rib units, beyond which the spleen can be judged as enlargement. On the cross-sectional images, the long axis of a normal spleen is not more than 15 cm, the transverse diameter is not more than 10 cm, and the thickness is not more than 6 cm (Fig. 2.9) [1, 3].

References

1. Jiang HC. Splenic surgery. Beijing: People's Military Medical Press; 2013.
2. Jiang HC. Splenic tumor surgery. Beijing: People's Military Medical Press; 2011.
3. Liu SW, Yang XF, Deng XF. Clinical anatomic series: abdominal. 2nd ed. Beijing: People's Health Press; 2014.
4. Liu SW, Liu C, Hu SY. Atlas of clinical anatomy of abdominal surgery. Jinan: Shandong Science and Technology Press; 2006.

5. Qiu FZ, Wang JB, Zhang HZ. Clinical anatomy of abdominal surgery. Jinan: Shandong Science and Technology Press; 2001.
6. Wu MC, Wu ZD. Huang Jiasi surgery. 7th ed. Beijing: People's Health Publishing House; 2008.
7. Xu JJ. The anatomic value of Chinese. 2nd ed. Beijing: People's Health Publishing House; 2014.
8. Richard LD, Vogl AW, Mitchell AWH, et al. Gray's atlas of anatomy. Philadelphia: Churchill Livingstone; 2008.
9. Skandalakis PN, Colborn GL, Skandalakis LJ, et al. The surgical anatomy of the spleen. Surg Clin North Am. 1993;73(4):747–68.
10. Chen XW, Han DB, Chen WP. Relationship between spleen and distant organs. Chin J Hepatobiliary Surg. 2005;11(5):359–60.

3 Pathology and Pathophysiology of Surgical Spleen Diseases

He Cai, Junhe Gou, Qijun Chen, and Bing Peng

3.1 Blood System Diseases

The function of spleen is closely related to the occurrence, development, and outcome of various blood system diseases. Splenectomy is also an effective method to treat or alleviate these diseases [1]. For hemolytic anemia diseases such as autoimmune hemolytic anemia (AIHA), hereditary spherocytosis, thalassemia, pyruvate kinase deficiency, and so on, spleen is the main place to destroy the abnormal red blood cells, and some selected patients could benefit from splenectomy; for hemorrhagic diseases such as immune thrombocytopenia (ITP), spleen is considered to be the main site of producing platelet-associated antibodies (PAIgG) and the main organ of platelet retention and destruction, and splenectomy as a second-line treatment can also achieve good results [2]; for malignant hematologic diseases such as Hodgkin's lymphoma, splenectomy is helpful for diagnosis and clinical stage. For primary lymphoma of the spleen as another example, such as follicular lymphoma, mantle cell lymphoma, and marginal area lymphoma, the 5-year survival rate can reach more than 30% via comprehensive treatment based on splenectomy [3]. In a word, spleen surgery is closely related to the clinical treatment of hematologic diseases. The following is a brief overview of the pathology and pathophysiology of spleen in AIHA, ITP, lymphoma, and other blood diseases.

3.1.1 Autoimmune Hemolytic Anemia

Autoimmune hemolytic anemia (AIHA) refers to production of antibody or complement on the surface of red blood cells due to the disorder of immune factors in patients, thus accelerating the destruction of red blood cells and leading to hemolytic anemia. When there is thrombocytopenia in the course of AIHA, it is called Evan's syndrome. The initiating factors of the disease are relatively complex, and in clinical practice, there is little knowledge about the pathophysiological process. However, according to the temperature required for the interaction between the antibody and the erythrocyte membrane, it can be divided into warm antibody type, cold antibody type, and mixed type. AIHA with warm antibody is normal, and mixed type is rare [4, 5]. The antibody of AIHA with warm antibody mainly belongs to IgG type, which is most active at 37 °C; the antibody of cold one mainly belongs to IgM type, which is most active at 20 °C. Although these two types of AIHA have different clinical char-

H. Cai · J. Gou · B. Peng (✉)
West China Hospital, Sichuan University, Chengdu, China

Q. Chen
West China Second University Hospital, Sichuan University, Chengdu, China

B. Peng (ed.), *Laparoscopic Surgery of the Spleen*, https://doi.org/10.1007/978-981-16-1216-9_3

acteristics, they also have something in common, including the shorter survival time of red blood cells in vivo, enhanced hematopoietic function of the bone marrow, and positive anti-human globulin test.

According to the etiology, warm antibody AIHA can be divided into two types: primary (50%) and secondary. The cause of primary AIHA, whose main clinical manifestation is hemolytic anemia, is unknown. Secondary AIHA is often secondary to lymphoproliferative diseases (20%), autoimmune diseases (20%), infection, and other tumors [6]. Cold antibody AIHA can be divided into cold agglutination syndrome and paroxysmal cold hemoglobinuria, and the latter is common in patients with syphilis, virus infection, and immune diseases. The mechanism of antibody production may be that the virus or other pathogenic factors act on the erythrocyte membrane and change the antigenicity of the membrane; the antibodies produced by some foreign antigens cross-react with the erythrocyte antigens; all kinds of reasons cause the normal immune system to be disordered and lose the ability to recognize the erythrocytes, thus producing abnormal autoantibodies. After the formation of autoantibodies, they can be adsorbed on the surface of red blood cells, or free in serum. According to different functions of the autoantibodies, it can be divided into complete antibody and incomplete antibody. Complete antibody can directly agglutinate or dissolve red blood cells, while incomplete antibody can sensitize red blood cells, making red blood cells phagocytized and destroyed by monocyte macrophage system. Incomplete antibodies are more common clinically [7, 8].

Autoantibodies IgG and/or complements (C3, C4) of the warm antibody AIHA directly cover the surface of red blood cells, making red blood cells agglutinate or dissolve (generally not in blood vessels). It can also make red blood cells adsorb on peripheral blood monocytes (usually the mega phagocytes in the spleen), which can wholly or partially phagocytize red blood cells or make red blood cells become rigid, and finally the red blood cells are destroyed in the spleen or other monocyte macrophage system. The cold antibodies are all IgM in cold agglutinin syndrome. At the temperature above 32 °C, the cold agglutinin does not react with red blood cells, and the optimal reaction temperature is 0–4 °C. At a low temperature, the concentration of cold agglutinin increases rapidly, and red blood cells agglutinate into large clots, colliding with each other in the circulatory system, resulting in mechanical damage. When the body temperature rises to 10–30 °C (the most appropriate temperature is 20–25 °C), hemolysis occurs. There is a kind of D-L antibody (7SIgG), which is also called "biphasic antibody" in the blood of patients with paroxysmal cold hemoglobinuria. The reason is that its hemolytic effect is the strongest when the body temperature drops to 0–4 °C and then rises immediately. When the temperature drops below 20 °C (preferably 15 °C), the D-L antibody can bind on the surface of red blood cells. The complement can promote the binding of this antibody, but the complement cannot be fully activated below 15 °C, and hemolysis does not occur. When the temperature rises to 37 °C, the activation of complement is completed, and hemolysis occurs [9].

First of all, we should find the cause of warm antibody AIHA and treat the primary disease. The first choice of medicine for medical treatment is adrenocortical hormone. Its mechanism is to inhibit the production of antibodies by lymphocytes, reduce the affinity between antibodies and erythrocytes, reduce the IgG and/or C3 receptors on macrophage membrane, and inhibit the binding ability of these receptors and erythrocytes membrane. Other medical treatments include immunosuppressive agents, cyclosporin A, intravenous injection of a large dose of gamma globulin, and blood transfusion. As the spleen is the main organ producing antibodies and the main place of destroying the sensitized red blood cells, the total effective rate of splenectomy on warm antibody AIHA is 60–75%, and the effect of IgG anti human globulin positive is the best, but due to the existence and effect of other medical treatment, the rate of splenectomy on warm antibody AIHA is low (10–20%) [10]. Although erythrocytes can be sensitized after splenectomy, the amount of antibody needed for sensitization increases by about ten times, and the effect on the life of erythrocytes decreases. After splenectomy, continuing to use glucocorticoid and other medical treatment can consolidate and improve the efficacy. The drug cannot be removed too early, so as to prevent recurrence [11].

The cold agglutinin syndrome lasts for a short time, and it is usually self-healed without using any medicine. Keeping warm is the main cure. Transfusion treatment should be given with more care, because the donor red blood cells are more vulnerable to cold agglutinin damage. Glucocorticoid and splenectomy are both ineffective. Patients with paroxysmal cold hemoglobinuria can often restore quickly due to hemolysis without special treatment. In order to prevent recurrence, it is mainly to keep warm and actively seek for treatment of primary disease. The effect of splenectomy is uncertain [12, 13].

The main morphological features of spleen in AIHA patients are macrophage proliferation and phagocytosis of macrophages to red blood cells. The spleen generally shows light to moderate enlargement (Fig. 3.1). It is hard, dark red, thin in capsule, and inconspicuous in splenic nodule. Its weight is between 14 and 1670 g, with an average of 650 g, which is 5.7 times the normal spleen weight. The spleen of AIHA with cold antibody is smaller than 400 g. Under the light microscope, the number of follicles in the spleen increases, the germinal center expands, the margin band widens, the spleen cord and the spleen sinuses are filled with red blood cells in varying degrees, and the phagocytosis of red blood cells in the sinuses is more prominent, while the spleen cord is lighter (Fig. 3.2). However, the white pulp of the patients treated with hormone has no germinal center, the spleen cord is full, and the spleen sinus is empty, which is very similar to spherocytosis. There is extramedullary hematopoiesis, sinus endothelium hyperplasia, macrophage proliferation, plasma cells, and hemosiderin deposition. By means of scanning electron microscopy, ultrathin sectioning, and freeze replica, the proliferation of macrophages in splenic sinuses, irregular shape, large amount of lysosomes and other organelles in cytoplasm, and many protuberances and microvilli on the surface are observed under transmission electron microscopy. There are many red cells adsorbed on the surface of macrophages, some of which have been partially or completely engulfed by macrophages. The macrophage process adsorption, capture, and phagocytosis can be seen. The spleen with Evian syndrome has the characteristics of hemolytic anemia and ITP, i.e., follicular hyperplasia, enlarged germinal center, more neutrophils in the red pulp, obvious hemosiderin deposition, wide distribution of iron staining-positive particles, and more extramedullary hematopoiesis.

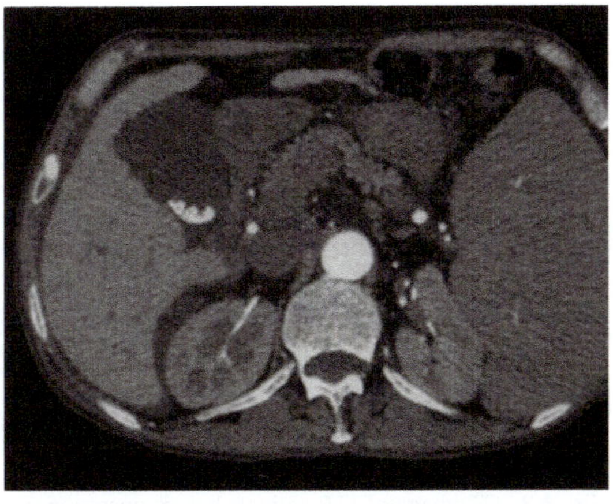

Fig. 3.1 CT of AIHA patients (spleen enlargement)

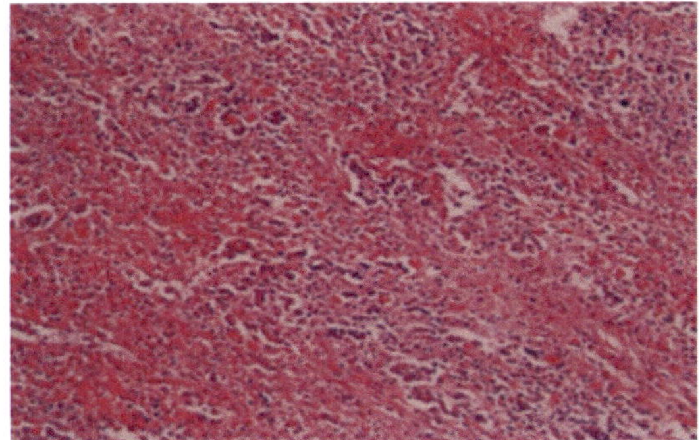

Fig. 3.2 HE staining light microscopy of spleen in AIHA patients

3.1.2 Immune Thrombocytopenic Purpura

ITP is a kind of acquired hemorrhagic disease with unknown causes. It can be divided into two types: primary and secondary. 80% of patients are primary ITP, which is currently considered to be related to immune disorders. For secondary ITP, the main method is to treat primary diseases, such as HIV and HCV. Most of them are self-limited diseases in children, while the spontaneous remission rate in adults is only 9% [11]. Clinically, it is characterized by thrombocytopenia, increase or normal number of megakaryocytes in bone marrow, and normal spleen size or slight enlargement of spleen.

At present, it is believed that the primary ITP is mainly mediated by immunity, that is, the imbalance of immune regulatory cells in the internal and external blood circulation of the spleen leads to the disorder of immune regulation; meanwhile, the spleen is the main place for the production of antiplatelet-related antibodies, and the IgG produced by the spleen of patients with chronic ITP is about seven times higher than that of the normal control spleen. Spleen tissue can synthesize IgG in vitro. IgG can also be washed from the spleen of patients with ITP. The monocyte macrophage system in the spleen can clear sensitized platelets, and the clearance rate is positively correlated with IgG content [14]. In addition, lymphocytes in the bone marrow of ITP patients can also produce platelet antibodies.

The antibodies act directly on the glycoprotein IIb/IIIa on the platelet membrane, and a few act on the glycoprotein Ib-IX complex. After the antibody-coated platelets are combined with the antigen-presenting cells and pass through the Fc receptor in the spleen, the platelets are destroyed, the life span of platelets is shortened, and the function is changed. The content of platelet-associated antibodies is negatively correlated with the life span of platelets. It is found that radioisotopes accumulated rapidly and massively in the spleen after transfusion of ^{51}Cr-labeled allogeneic platelets to ITP patients and scanning of the spleen. The body surface count of ^{111}In-oxine-labeled platelets also shows that platelets are mainly suppressed and eliminated in the spleen [15].

The spleen not only produces antiplatelet antibodies and macrophages but also provides an environment where platelets are easy to combine with antibodies. It is the main organ that destroys and detains platelets [16]. The first-line treatment is mainly applying glucocorticoid and immunoglobulin, but in European and American countries, anti-D antibody is also administered to the patients; splenectomy is the second-line treatment for ITP, which is helpful to improve the immune regulatory status and reduce platelet damage. In most patients, platelets increase to 100 × 10^9/L within 1 week after splenectomy, and in a few patients, it takes several months to normalize platelets. In general, the effective rate of splenectomy in the treatment of ITP is 70–90%, but the recurrence rate is 9.6–22.7%. 60–80% of the patients recover after the platelet recovery, but it is ineffective for 5–20% of the patients [17, 18]. Because the spleen usually remains in normal size or slightly enlarged, laparoscopic splenectomy is very suitable for ITP [19, 20]. Retrospective study shows that laparoscopic splenectomy allows patients to have less pain, quicker recovery, and shorter hospital stay [21, 22].

The spleen in ITP looks normal or slightly enlarged (Fig. 3.3), the number and the size of follicles increase, the number of lobulated leukocytes and nuclear fragments in red pulp increases, and the iron staining is negative for those with no hemosiderin. The number of phagocytes in splenic cord increases, and the cytoplasm contains a large number of secondary lysosomes (Fig. 3.4).

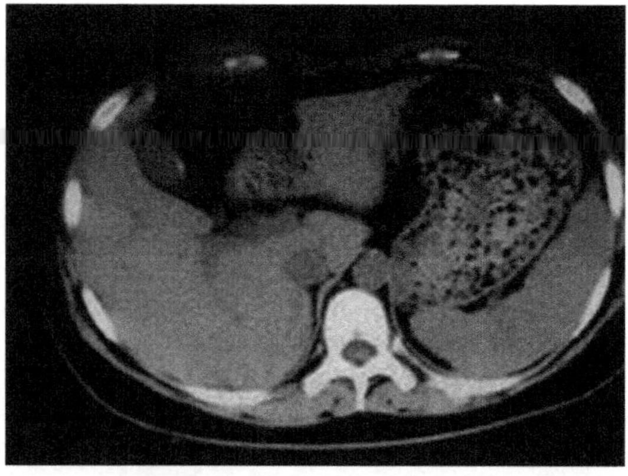

Fig. 3.3 CT image of ITP patients before operation (the same as normal spleen)

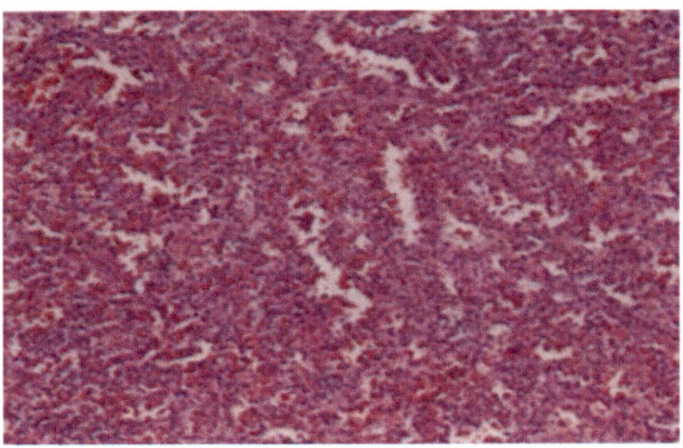

Fig. 3.4 HE staining light microscopy of spleen in ITP patients (×200)

3.1.3 Lymphoma

As the largest immune organ and blood filtering organ in the body, spleen is often affected by systemic diseases such as lymphoma and leukemia. In the past, open splenectomy was an important means to facilitate the diagnosis and staging of Hodgkin's lymphoma, and it was the key to determine the best treatment for patients: generally only patients above the diaphragm were involved in radiotherapy, while other patients received radiotherapy plus chemotherapy [23, 24]. However, with the progress in the imaging technology, especially the application of PET-CT imaging technology, $^{[18]}$F-FDG PET/CT imaging uses the principle that the glucose metabolism rate of tumor cells increases, and the faster tumor cells proliferate, the more glucose they ingest, to observe the cell function and metabolic activity at the molecular level; generally, tumor cells with positive response to chemotherapy show the decrease, delay, or stop of tumor cell metabolism activity after chemotherapy, and PET/CT imaging shows the decrease or no ingestion of $^{[18]}$F-FDG. Therefore, PET/CT can accurately reflect the treatment effect, without waiting for weeks or months to determine the effect of tumor volume changes, which changes the traditional imaging technology (such as B-ultrasound, CT, and MRI technology) based on the morphological changes of lesions to assess the treatment effect of lymphoma. PET/CT can change the stage and treatment plan of patients with Hodgkin's lymphoma, improve the accuracy of treatment, and have a positive impact on the prognosis of patients. Combined with the improvement of the treatment strategy, the combination treatment replaces the treatment mode of over-expanding the radiation site. After treatment, PET/CT status can be used to assess the treatment effect, which is helpful to develop individualized treatment plan. It makes the surgical staging and splenectomy less commonly used in the treatment of Hodgkin's lymphoma [25–27]. After treatment, PET/CT status can be used to assess the therapeutic effect and help to make individualized treatment plan. Laparoscopic splenectomy significantly reduces operative trauma and complications, even when surgical staging is required.

Primary splenic lymphoma is rarely seen in clinical practices (Fig. 3.5), which mainly refers to the lesions in the spleen and hilus lymph nodes. At the same time, a small number of abdominal lymph nodes, bone marrow, and liver can be involved, but there is no superficial lymph node swelling, which is currently considered to be closely related to virus infection [28]. Most of the pathological types are non-Hodgkin's lymphoma (NHL), with B cell being the main source, including many subtypes such as follicular lymphoma, marginal zone lymphoma, mantle cell lymphoma, small cell lymphoma, and diffuse large B-cell lymphoma (Fig. 3.6). Marginal zone lymphoma, follicular lymphoma, and small lym-

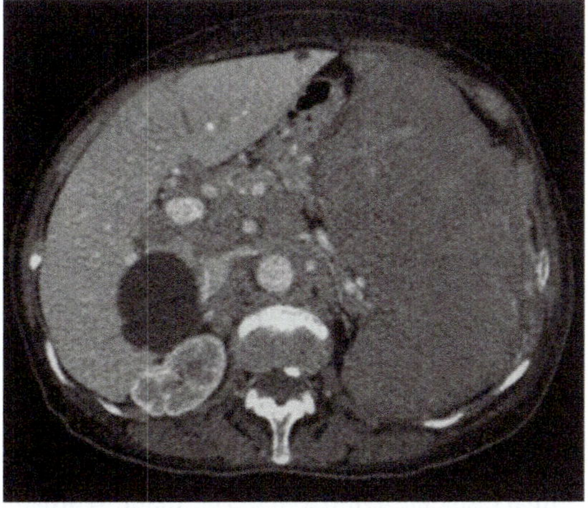

Fig. 3.5 CT of primary splenic lymphoma (diffuse large B lymphoma)

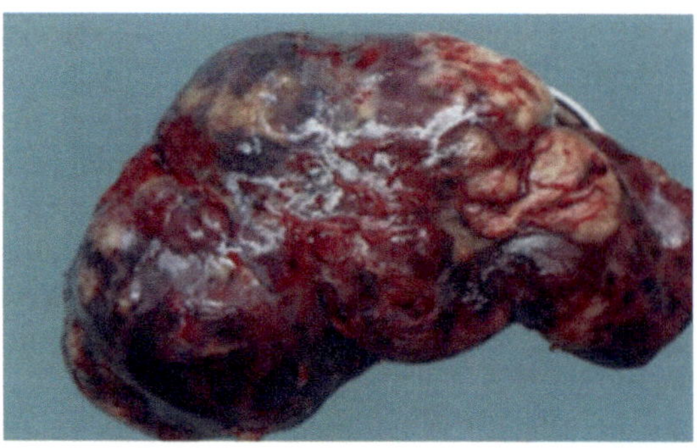

Fig. 3.6 Postoperative diagram of primary splenic lymphoma (diffuse large B lymphoma)

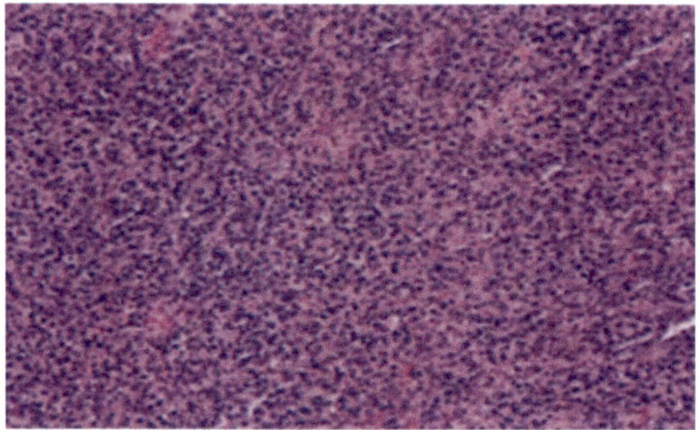

Fig. 3.7 HE staining light microscopy of patients with primary splenic lymphoma (diffuse large B lymphoma) (×200)

phoid lymphoma are usually classified as inert lymphoma, mantle cell lymphoma, and diffuse large B lymphoma which are invasive lymphoma (Fig. 3.7), and the disease progresses rapidly and is highly invasive. T-cell lymphoma is mainly peripheral T-cell lymphoma [29].

According to Ahman's staging [30], the primary splenic lymphoma is divided into three stages. This staging method has certain guiding significance for the comprehensive surgical treatment. Stage I tumor is completely limited in the spleen, not involving the splenic hilar lymph nodes and distant organs; stage II tumor involves the splenic hilar lymph nodes; stage III has distant invasion such as the liver, celiac lymph nodes, and even bone marrow. At present, there is no unified diagnosis and treatment guideline for primary splenic lymphoma. The main treatment is still splenectomy combined with local radiotherapy, systemic chemotherapy, and targeted treatment. Among them, early diagnosis and comprehensive treatment are the key elements.

The prognosis factors are related to pathology, typing and treatment, mainly pathology, and classification. For the mildly and moderately malignant types, the 3-year and 5-year survival rates are 75% and 60%, respectively, while for the highly malignant type, the 3-year survival rate is 20% [31]. The 2-year and 5-year survival rates are 71% and 43%, respectively, in patients with stage I primary splenic lymphoma and 21% and 14%, respectively, in patients with stage III. Most scholars believe that the prognosis of stage I and stage II patients with primary splenic lymphoma is similar to that of other stage I NHL, while that of stage III patients is the same as that of other stage IV NHL [32].

3.2 Portal Hypertension

Portal hypertension (PH) is a syndrome caused by abnormal hemodynamics of portal vein system and prolonged increase of pressure due to liver cirrhosis, obstruction of main portal vein or hepatic vein, etc. The normal free portal vein pressure ranges from 9.5 to 17.6 mmHg (13–24 cmH_2O), with an average of 13.2 mmHg (18 cmH_2O). The difference between hepatic vein wedge pressure and hepatic vein free pressure is the hepatic venous pressure gradient (HVPG). HVPG applied to represent portal vein pressure has become a recognized gold standard, but it is only suitable for patients with sinusoidal portal hypertension mainly caused by hepatitis cirrhosis or alcoholic cirrhosis. The normal value range of HVPG is 0–5 mmHg. When HVPG reaches 10 mmHg or above, it indicates the existence of clinically significant portal hypertension [33]. At present, according to the location of blood flow obstruction, PH is divided into presinusoidal and post-sinusoidal. Presinusoidal portal hypertension includes extrahepatic (portal vein obstruction, increase of splenic blood flow, etc.) or intrahepatic (tumor infiltration and poisoning in portal area), and post-sinusoidal portal hypertension includes hepatic vein obstruction and circulatory failure. Intrahepatic sinusoidal PH with cirrhosis is the most common [34].

In normal case, the splenic vein blood flow accounts for 20–40% of the total portal vein blood flow. The increase in the pressure of the portal vein directly leads to the stagnation of blood flow in the splenic vein, which makes the spleen congestive with or without hypersplenism. At this time, the splenic vein blood flow can be as high as 60% of the portal vein blood flow. Due to the poor drainage of the portal vein, the spleen is hyperemic, but there is no correlation between the size of the spleen and the pressure of the portal vein. The enlargement of spleen, in turn, further increases the blood flow of portal vein, aggravates the high dynamic perfusion of portal vein system, and further increases the pressure of portal vein [35]. Due to the circuitous blood epidemic path, the retention time can be as long as 1 h, resulting in the increase in mechanical damage of blood cells, which is manifested as hypersplenism, leukopenia, thrombocytopenia, and hyperplastic anemia.

The most important collateral circulation opening in esophageal and gastric fundus varices caused by PH includes left gastric vein, short gastric vein, and posterior gastric vein (Fig. 3.8). The anterior branch of the left gastric vein penetrates the gastric wall 2–3 cm below the gastroesophageal junction and is divided into the submucosal branches of the cardia. These branches are connected with the esophageal varices in the lower part of the esophagus, and the posterior branch mainly supplies blood to the paraesophageal varices.

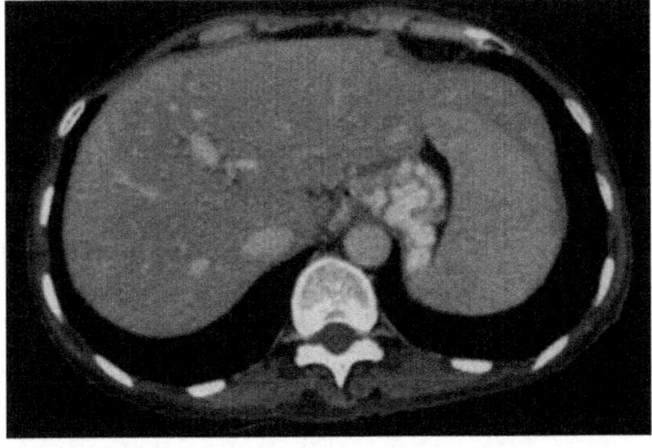

Fig. 3.8 CT of esophageal and gastric fundus varices in patients with portal hypertension

Under physiological conditions, 3–5 short gastric veins flow to the splenic vein inside the spleen along the gastric fundus and left great curvature side. In PH patients, the splenic vein flows into the gastric fundus through the short gastric vein. In most cases, the splenic vein flows into the superior vena cava through the esophageal varices, and in few cases, it flows into the inferior vena cava through the left renal vein. The posterior gastric vein is a unique blood vessel communicating branch that collects the gastric fundus and is different from the left and short gastric veins. It is difficult to find it under physiological conditions. In about 42% of PH patients, the posterior gastric vein supplies blood to the varicose vein of the gastric fundus. Similarly, in most cases, it flows into the superior vena cava through the varicose vein of the esophagus, and in few cases, it enters the inferior vena cava through the left renal vein communicating tributary [36, 37]. In some cases, it also passes through the spleen-stomach-diaphragm-adrenal gland-renal vein shunt, which increases the risk of bleeding due to the long distance and high resistance [38]. Of course, the shunt of spleen and kidney or gastrorenal vein will increase the risk of hepatic encephalopathy [39]. In addition, some unusual collateral circulation can lead to heterotopic varices such as duodenum, jejunum, ileum, colon, anorectum, and retroperitoneal varices. The clinical treatment effect of different open collateral circulation of digestive tract varices may vary greatly. Zhao et al. [40] found that when 86 patients with endoscopic diagnosis of esophagogastric varices were scanned with spiral CT, it was found that 32.56% (28/86) of the varices were supplied by a single left gastric vein, and 30.23% (26/86) were mainly supplied by a short gastric vein at the distal end of the spleen/posterior gastric vein. Therefore, embolization or disconnection of gastric coronary vein is not effective for the patients with short stomach and posterior gastric vein whose blood supply vessel is the distal part of the spleen, while it is effective for the patients whose blood supply is mainly from the gastric coronary vein, so an accurate assessment should be made before operation [41].

The principles of treatment for PH patients are early, continuous, and lifelong treatment. The surgical operation for PH patients developed in the 1940s–1960s and even in the 1970s was the only effective way to treat PH esophagogastric variceal bleeding. However, later studies found that the prognosis of PH patients was mainly determined by the liver function itself. With the progress in endoscopy and interventional technology, "drug-endoscopy-interventional" treatment was the main means of treatment of PH patients, and liver transplantation was the final means [42, 43]; although, compared with endoscopic therapy, surgery has a lower rate of postoperative rebleeding, its role in PH patients is controversial. Various guidelines provide different experiences in the indication of applied surgery and the status of surgery. The choice of operation mode is also affected by doctor's experience, liver transplantation, and other factors, but the mainstream operation mode includes various devascularization and distal splenorenal shunt (DSRS) [44, 45]. The purpose of surgical treatment is mainly to solve the rupture and bleeding caused by esophageal and gastric fundus varices and then to solve the splenomegaly and hypersplenism. After splenectomy, the blood flow of splenic vein, which accounts for 60% of the total blood flow of portal vein, is reduced. At the same time, the operation does not change the direction of portal vein to hepatic blood flow, but keeps the blood flow of portal vein at a normal high level. It could delay the development of PH, reduce the probability of bleeding caused by esophageal and gastric fundus varices rupture, and eliminate hypersplenism of spleen function [46]. Minimally invasive surgery is one of the development directions of surgical technology. Laparoscopic technology has profoundly changed the surgical operation at the technical level. More and more laparoscopic devascularization operations have been carried out gradually, and shunt operations have also been reported. Correct selection of surgical indications and experienced endoscopic surgeons is also an important factor to ensure the safety and effectiveness for performing laparoscopic splenectomy (Fig. 3.9) or hand-assisted surgery in such patients (even megalosplenia). Meanwhile, laparoscopic splenectomy has the advantages of less intraoperative bleeding and quick postoperative recovery. The application of laparoscopic technology in PH surgery may be the future development direction, but more clinical evidence is needed [47, 48].

In general, the weight of spleen can reach 500–1000 g, even 5000 g. The texture is solid, the capsule is thickened, the trabecula is thickened, and the fibrosis is serious. The section is dark red and flat, and the white pulp is reduced. Sometimes there are small iron spots in grayish yellow or yellowish brown on the section, which are called tobacco flakes, i.e., Gandy-Gamna nodules. Under the light microscope, the fibrous scar tissue with iron and calcium salt deposition is found (Fig. 3.10).

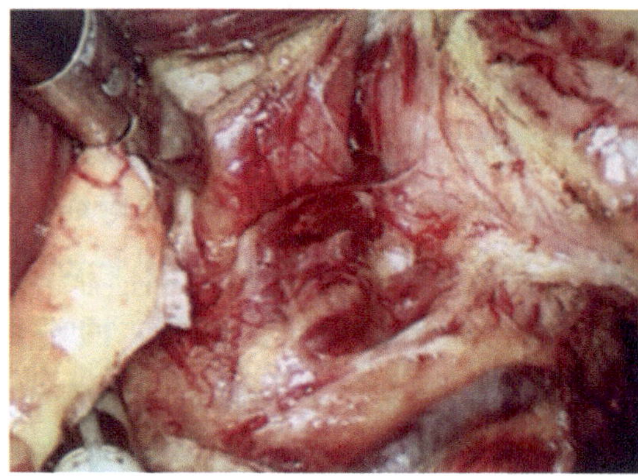

Fig. 3.9 Varicose lower esophageal vein after the laparoscopic devascularization operation

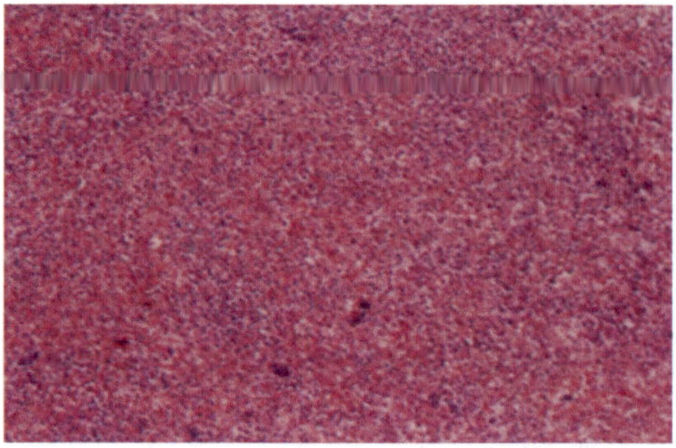

Fig. 3.10 HE staining light microscopy of splenectomy specimen of patients with portal hypertension (×200)

3.3 Splenic Space-Occupying Lesion

Splenic space-occupying lesions include primary and secondary lesions. Primary space-occupying lesions refer to spleen cyst, benign tumor, and malignant tumor. The incidence of benign tumors in the spleen is about 0.14%, and the incidence of malignant tumors is no more than 0.64% of all malignant tumors [49]. The occult onset of the disease can occur at any age, and the proportion of men and women is equal. The most common primary benign tumors include cysts, hemangiomas, lymphangiomas, hamartomas, and so on. The most common primary malignant tumors include lymphoma, angiosarcoma, vascular endothelial sarcoma, and so on. Malignant lymphoma is often accompanied by systemic symptoms, such as fever and fatigue, which features short course and fast progress, often complicated with symptoms of hypersplenism, such as anemia and thrombocytopenia.

Secondary splenic space-occupying lesions are dominated by metastasis. The diagnosis should be based on the patient's medical history, symptoms, physical signs, laboratory examination, and imaging examination results [50]. Generally, the clinical diagnosis is difficult and depends on B-ultrasound, CT, MRI, and other imaging examinations (Fig. 3.11). However, surgical resection of spleen mass is still needed for pathological section diagnosis. B-ultrasound is of great significance in the screening of splenic tumors. It is reported in the literature at home and abroad that the localization rate of B-ultrasound for splenic space-occupying lesions is close to 100%, but it is of little value in qualitative diagnosis of benign and malignant splenic lesions. Abdominal CT is superior to B-ultrasound in both location and qualitative diagnosis of splenic lesions. In particular, enhanced CT has an important clinical application value in distinguishing tumor neovascularization. MRI is similar to CT in the detection rate of splenic space-occupying lesions, but the former has advantages in understanding the blood supply of tumor [51].

3.3.1 Splenic Cyst

Splenic cyst belongs to benign a space-occupying lesion. It can be divided into true cyst and false cyst according to the pathological tissue structure. True cysts include inclusion cysts, epidermoid cysts, lymphangiocysts, vascular cysts, and parasitic cysts. The inner wall of cysts is lined with one or more layers of cells or squamous epithelium, glandular epithelium, vascular epithelium, or lymphangioepithelium (Fig. 3.12). Pseudocysts are more common in young men. Most of the cysts are under the splenic capsule. The wall of the cysts is composed of fibrous tissue. There are no epithelia on the inner wall. Necrotic tissue and old blood fluid or serous fluid is found in the cysts. The common causes include trauma and specific (such as tuberculosis) or nonspecific inflammation. Ultrasound testing results show a well-defined cystic space, clear boundary,

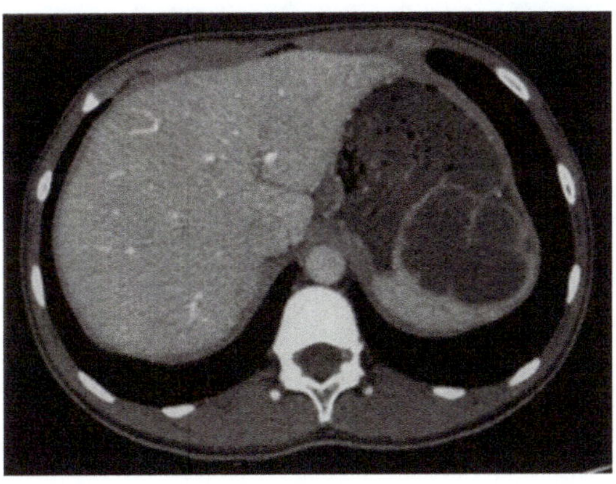

Fig. 3.11 CT of spleen cyst

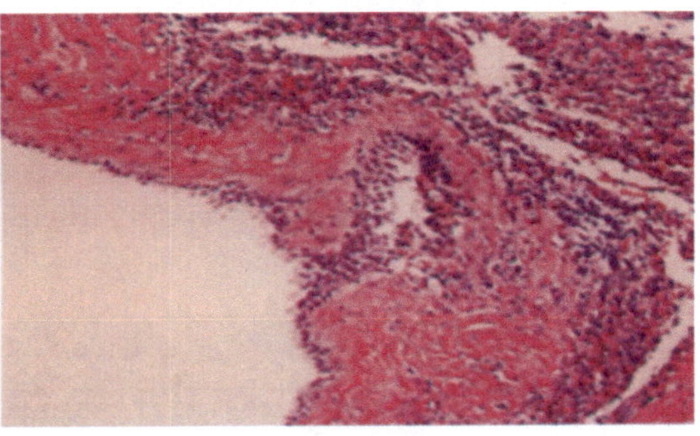

Fig. 3.12 HE staining light microscopy of spleen showing benign cyst, lined with single cuboid or flat epithelium

and separation in some patients, without echoic dark area and blood flow signal in the cyst [52].

It is generally believed that no surgical treatment is needed for epithelial cysts and pseudocysts smaller than 4 cm and those without symptoms, while for cysts larger than 5 cm, there is a risk of rupture and bleeding reported in the literature. The treatment can be performed by cyst extraction, incision and drainage, partial splenectomy, or splenectomy (Fig. 3.13). In recent years, according to the recognition of spleen function, according to the location, size, surrounding anatomical structure, and the relationship with splenic portal vessels, laparoscopic partial splenectomy may be a better choice [53].

3.3.2 Hemangioma of Spleen

Most of splenic hemangiomas are cavernous hemangiomas. There are also reports of capillary hemangiomas and venous hemangiomas. Most of them are found by physical examination, rarely causing splenomegaly, but they can be complicated with splenic infarction, infection, and calcification, with a few causing malignant transformation. B-mode ultrasonography shows inhomogeneous or nodular hypoechoic changes in splenic parenchyma. There may be scar formation in the center of hemangioma, which shows lower density under CT or high density with hemorrhage (Fig. 3.14). Because of the existence of scar tissue and thrombus in the center, the blood flow is slow, and there is no enhanced area in the center of the focus in the delayed period. Therefore, delayed scanning to observe the hemodynamic characteristics of the mass is of great value in the diagnosis of hemangioma [54]. Small and asymptomatic hemangiomas with definite diagnosis need not be treated. They need close follow-up and regular reexamination. For large hemangiomas growing under observation, splenectomy or partial splenectomy is feasible (Fig. 3.15), while laparoscopic surgery is more advantageous [55].

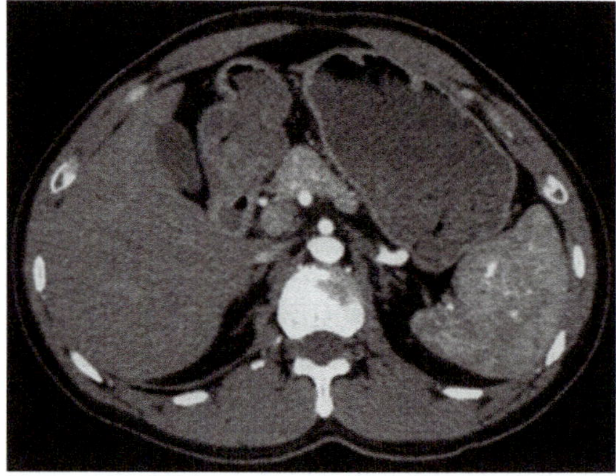

Fig. 3.14 Enhanced CT of splenic hemangioma

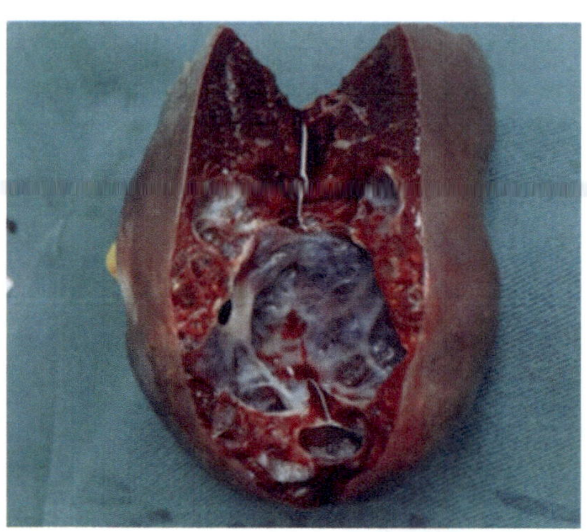

Fig. 3.13 Section of spleen cyst after laparoscopic partial splenectomy

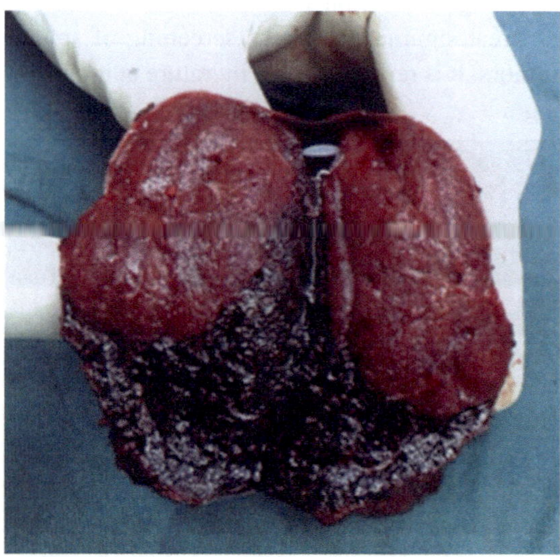

Fig. 3.15 Section of splenic hemangioma after laparoscopic partial splenectomy

In addition, the splenic sinus littoral cell hemangioma is a rare splenic angiogenic tumor. Its pathological features are as follows: nodular protuberances on the surface of the spleen are generally seen, which are not glossy; there are more gray-brown brittle nodules on the section, with a diameter of 0.2–1.0 cm, with clear boundary, but without capsule. Under the light microscope, the lesions are nodular in different sizes, located between the red pulp and the surrounding spleen tissue. The nodules are composed of a large number of irregular dilated sinusoid like cavities, which are generally wider than the normal splenic sinuses. A few of them are dilated into sacs; some of them are papillary and protruded into the lumen. Their axes are fibrous stroma, and the lumen wall is lined with monolayer endothelial cells. In part of the dilated vascular space, exfoliated endothelial cells can be seen, and lymphocytes, plasma cells, and a small number of neutrophils are scattered in the stroma (Fig. 3.16).

3.3.3 Splenic Metastasis

Metastatic tumors of the spleen are mostly malignant tumors derived from the epithelial system, such as skin cancer, breast cancer, ovarian cancer (Fig. 3.17), and lung cancer, which are relatively rare. Most of the metastasis ways are mainly blood circulation, and the lymphatic pathway is rare. There are also adjacent organ cancers invading the planting. It is often considered that there are multiple organ metastases in the whole body when spleen metastasis occurs [56]. Some studies have pointed out that malignant lymphoma is the most common invasion of the spleen. 30–40% of Hodgkin's lymphoma and 10–40% of non-Hodgkin's lymphoma have splenic metastasis [57]. In addition to ovarian cancer and solitary splenic metastasis, the treatment is mainly palliative and symptomatic because of its late cancer performance and poor prognosis. For patients with ovarian cancer, we should strive to remove the primary tumor reduction and splenectomy, because it can eliminate the immune negative effect of the spleen in late stage cancer and has a good effect (Fig. 3.18).

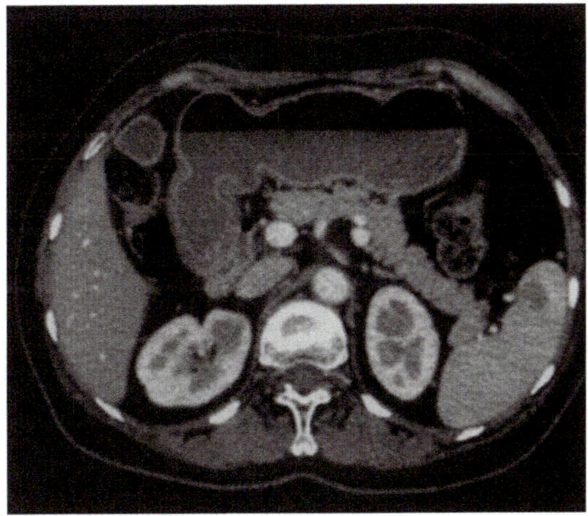

Fig. 3.17 Ovarian serous adenocarcinoma with lymph node metastasis of spleen and hilus

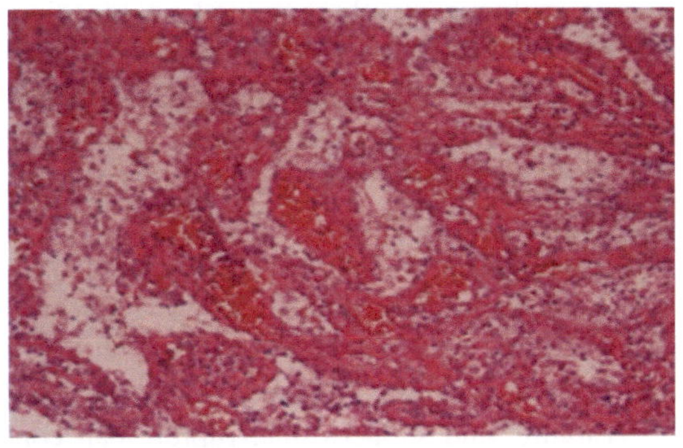

Fig. 3.16 HE staining light microscopy of splenic sinus littoral cell hemangioma

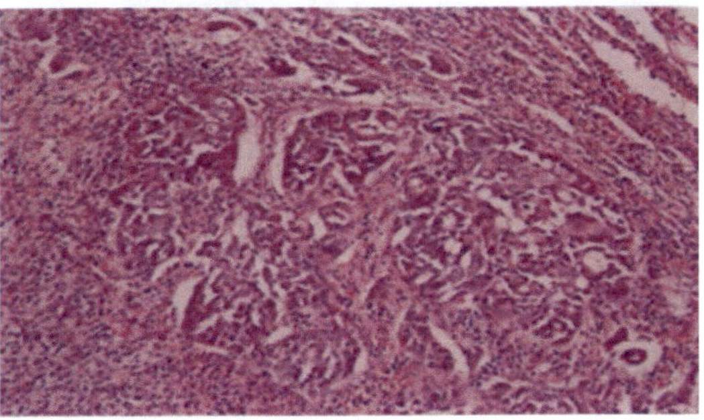

Fig. 3.18 HE staining light microscopy of ovarian serous adenocarcinoma with lymph node metastasis of spleen and hilus

3.4 Traumatic Splenic Rupture

Spleen is one of the most vulnerable organs among abdominal organs. For example, the spleen with pathological changes (portal hypertension, schistosomiasis, lymphoma, etc.) is more likely to damage and rupture. The incidence of spleen injury can be as high as 40–50% in various abdominal traumas, which is relatively common in clinical practices. According to the different injury factors, the traumatic spleen injury can be divided into two types, open spleen injury and closed spleen injury:

(a) Open spleen injury: mostly caused by stab, bullet penetration, and explosion, often combined with other organ injury
(b) Closed spleen injury: mostly occurring in traffic accidents, followed by fall injury, left chest injury, and left upper abdomen contusion

According to the history of trauma, clinical manifestations, and the results of abdominal puncture, the diagnostic rate is as high as 90%. B-ultrasound, CT, and other imaging examinations are helpful for further diagnosis, and dynamic observation of the degree and scope of spleen injury, especially CT examination (Fig. 3.19), can be used as the gold standard for diagnosis [58]. At the same time, these objective indicators are of great significance for clinical typing and classification, treatment plan formulation, and efficacy assessment.

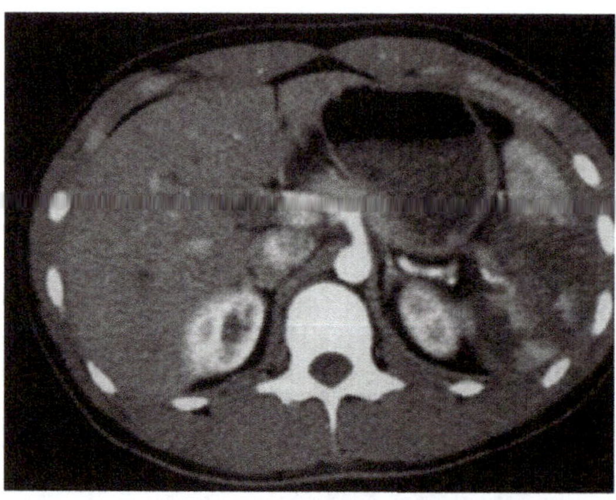

Fig. 3.19 Enhanced CT of traumatic splenic rupture

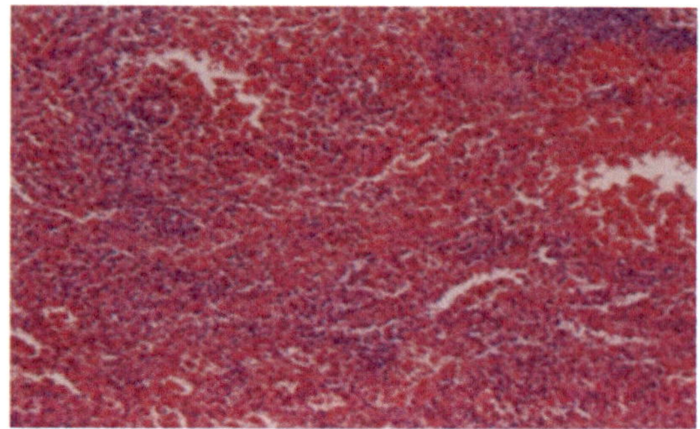

Fig. 3.20 HE staining light microscopy of spleen trauma

Most of the ruptures of the spleen run along the edge of the splenic segment (Fig. 3.20). Most of the damages do not involve the major blood vessels of the splenic hilum. If the rupture is along the direction of the splenic segment, there are few ruptures of the splenic segment blood vessels, with slow bleeding and short duration. If the rupture crosses the spleen, the blood vessels are damaged seriously, the amount of bleeding is large, and the duration is long. If the injury of splenic pedicle and hilum is involved, a large amount of bleeding will occur in a short time, resulting in hemorrhagic shock and life-threatening. According to the types of injury, it can be divided into central rupture, subperiosteal rupture, true rupture, and delayed rupture:

(a) Central rupture: central rupture of spleen parenchyma, mostly showing local bleeding, often without clear bleeding manifestations.
(b) Subperiosteal rupture: subperiosteal parenchyma rupture of spleen, but the peritoneum remaining intact, mostly showing tension hematoma formed under the capsule.
(c) True rupture: spleen parenchyma and peritoneum rupture at the same time, with typical intraperitoneal bleeding manifestations.
(d) Delayed rupture: delayed rupture, central rupture, and subperiosteal rupture can con-

tinue to develop, leading to the expansion of parenchymal and subperiosteal rupture, which is called true rupture.

At the Sixth National Symposium on Spleen Surgery, we discussed and passed the "grading of spleen injury":

Grade I subperiosteal rupture of spleen or slight injury of capsule and parenchyma, with the length of splenic laceration seen in operation ≤5.0 cm and depth ≤1.0 cm

Grade II total length of splenic laceration >5.0 cm, depth >1.0 cm, but splenic hilum is not involved, or splenic segment blood vessels are involved

Grade III splenic rupture and splenic laceration, or damage of blood vessels of splenic lobes

Grade IV extensive rupture of the spleen or damage of the splenic pedicle and the main artery and vein [59]

Based on the principle of "life first, spleen second," the treatment strategy adopts the individualized treatment. Mild injury can be treated conservatively, while severe injury needs timely and effective surgical treatment. The way of surgical treatment needs to be selected according to the general condition of patients, the type and degree of spleen injury, and the combined injury. Generally, there are four grades of treatment: Grade I, non-surgical treatment, agglutination, and coagulation hemostasis, suture repair; Grade II, suture repair, partial splenectomy, rupture, and bundling, ligation of splenic artery; Grade III, partial splenectomy, ligation of splenic artery; and Grade IV, total splenectomy + transplantation of splenic tissue.

In recent years, with the promotion of laparoscopic technique, it has also been used in patients with traumatic splenic rupture, but there is no unified standard. Generally, laparoscopic surgery can be chosen for the following patients [60, 61]: (a) children or young patients; (b) patients with stable hemodynamics or those with stable hemodynamics after infusion and transfusion; (c) patients with less severe abdominal pain and less obvious signs of peritonitis; (d) patients with spleen injury, but without serious multiple injury (such as chest injury, spine, pelvis, and limb fracture) that may affect the selection and change of body position during operation, and with light spleen injury as showed via B Ultrasound or CT examination; (e) patients with delayed spleen rupture; and (f) patients with spleen injury within grade III as showed via the imaging examination. Open surgery may be chosen without hesitation for the following patients: (a) patients with unstable hemodynamics, or those still with unstable hemodynamics after active anti shock treatment; (b) patients with more serious cavity organ rupture and high occurrence of abdominal infection and rebleeding after the surgery; (c) patients with multiple injuries such as liver rupture, brain injury, and chest injury; (d) patients with severe Grade III or Grade IV splenic trauma, such as splenic pedicle avulsion, rupture of splenic artery and vein trunk, severe and extensive splenic contusion, and hemorrhage; (e) patients with pathological splenic injury; and (f) patients with other organ diseases and unable to tolerate laparoscopic surgery. However, for patients who cannot be assessed whether the spleen is damaged or not and the extent of the injury before operation, the choice of laparotomy may increase unnecessary trauma. At this time, the choice of laparoscopic exploration and treatment can better solve this problem. Therefore, as long as the patients are properly selected and the indications of operation are correctly grasped, the application of laparoscopic technique in traumatic splenic rupture is safe and feasible [62]. For patients with the above indications, if the spleen injury only involves the upper or lower pole of the spleen (the degree of spleen injury is Grade II or Grade III), laparoscopic partial splenectomy (Fig. 3.21) is also safe and feasible [63].

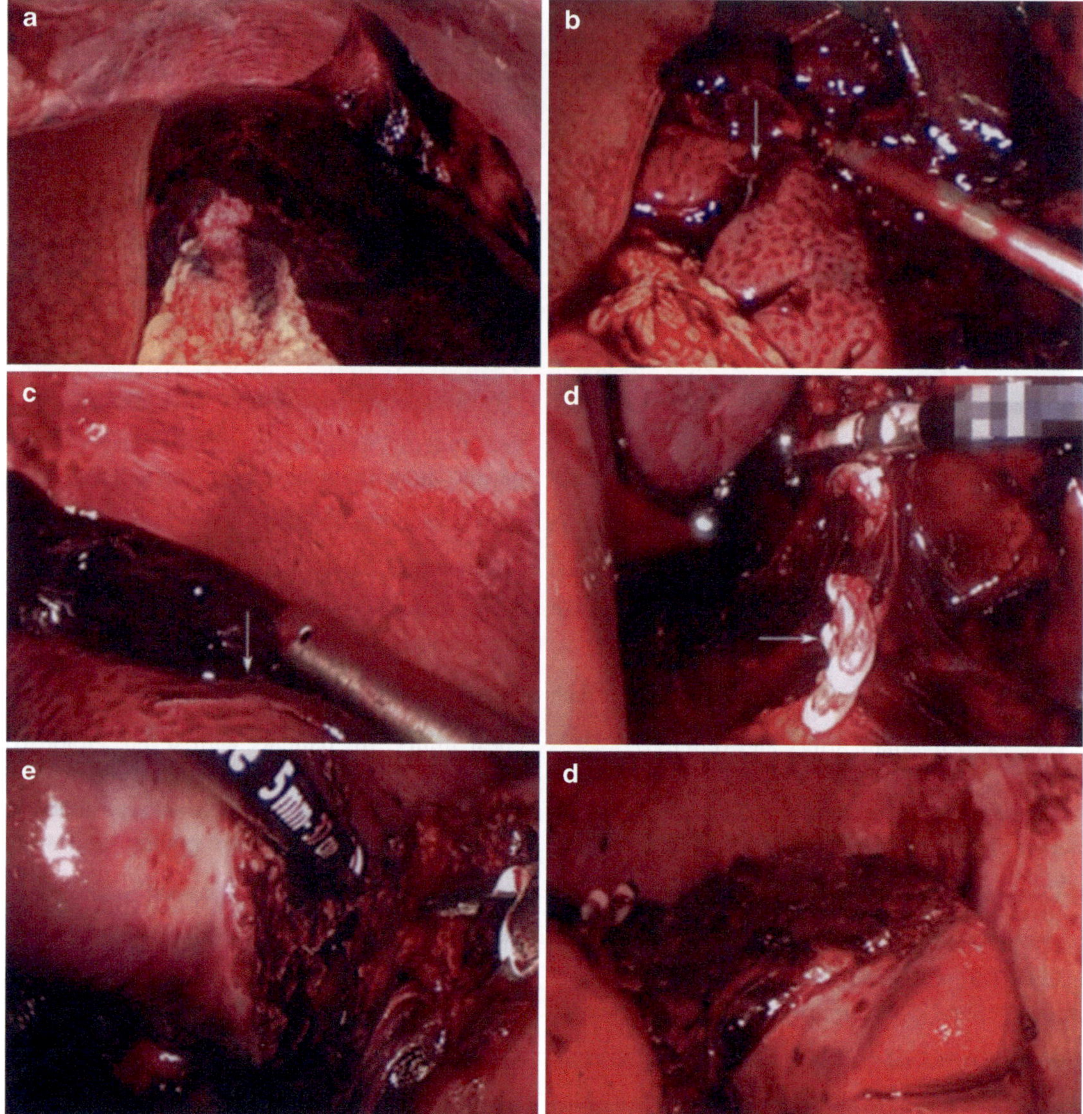

Fig. 3.21 Laparoscopic partial splenectomy for traumatic spleen. (**a**) Large peritoneal hematocele around the spleen; (**b**) surface rupture of the spleen (white arrow); (**c**) posterior rupture of the spleen (white arrow); (**d**) ligation of splenic artery branches; (**e**) dissection of spleen parenchyma with LigaSure; (**f**) incisal edge of laparoscopic partial splenectomy

References

1. Schwartz SI. Role of splenectomy in hematologic disorders. World J Surg. 1996;20(9):1156–9.
2. Ding XJ, Shen D, Lin BJ, et al. Practical hematology. Shanghai: Shanghai Medical University Press; 1992.
3. Greenberg PL, Steed SM. Splenic granulocytopoiesis and production of colony-stimulating activity in lymphoma and leukemia. Blood. 1981;57(1):119–29.
4. Aladjidi N, Leverger G, Leblanc T, et al. New insights into childhood autoimmune hemolytic anemia: a French national observational study of 265 children. Haematologica. 2011;96(5):655–63.
5. Genty I, Michel M, Hermine O, et al. Characteristics of autoimmune hemolytic anemia in adults: retrospective analysis of 83 cases. Rev Med Interne. 2002;23(11):901–9.
6. Barcellini W, Fattizzo B, Zaninoni A, et al. Clinical heterogeneity and predictors of outcome in primary

autoimmune hemolytic anemia: a GIMEMA study of 308 patients. Blood. 2014;124(19):2930–6.
7. Crosby WH, Rappaport H. Autoimmune hemolytic anemia. I. Analysis of hematologic observations with particular reference to their prognostk value. A survey of 57 cases. Blood. 1957;12(1):42–55.
8. Snowden JA, Saccardi R, Allez M, et al. Haematopoietic SCT in severe autoimmune diseases: updated guidelines of the European Group for blood and marrow transplantation. Bone Marrow Transplant. 2012;47(6):770–90.
9. Mauro FR, Foa R, Cerretti R, et al. Autoimmune hemolytic anemia in chronic lymphocytic leukemia: clinical, therapeutic, and prognostic features. Blood. 2000;95(9):2786–92.
10. Berentsen S, How I. manage cold agglutinin disease. Br J Haematol. 2011;153(3):309–17.
11. Lambert MP, Gernsheimer TB. Clinical updates in adult immune thrombocytopenia. Blood. 2017;129(21):2829–35.
12. Berentsen S, Randen U, Vågan AM, et al. High response rate and durable remissions following fludarabine and rituximab combination therapy for chronic cold agglutinin disease. Blood. 2010;116(17):3180.
13. Swiecicki PL, Hegerova LT, Gertz MA. Cold agglutinin disease. Blood. 2013;122(7):1114–21.
14. George JN, Woolf SH, Raskob GE, et al. Idiopathic thrombocytopenic purpura: a practice guideline developed by explicit methods for the American Society of Hematology. Blood. 1996;88(1):3–40.
15. Cines DB, Cuker A, Semple JW. Pathogenesis of immune thrombocytopenia. Presse Med. 2014;43(4):49–59.
16. Nieswandt B, Bergmeier W, Rackebrandt K. Identification of critical antigen-specific mechanisms in the development of immune thrombocytopenic purpura in mice. Blood. 2000;96(7):2520–7.
17. Fogarty PF. Chronic immune thrombocytopenia in adults: epidemiology and clinical presentation. Hematol Oncol Clin North Am. 2009;23(6):1213–21.
18. Umar S, Diehn FE, Gertz MA, et al. Splenectomy for immune thrombocytopenic purpura: long-term results and treatment of postsplenectomy relapses. Ann Hematol. 2002;81(6):312–9.
19. Hmed R, Devasia AJ, Viswabandya A, et al. Long-term outcome following splenectomy for chronic and persistent immune thrombocytopenia (ITP) in adults and children: splenectomy in ITP. Ann Hematol. 2016;95(9):1429–34.
20. Guan Y, Wang S, Xue F, et al. Long-term results of splenectomy in adult chronic immune thrombocytopenia. Eur J Haematol. 2017;98(3):235–41.
21. Wang X, Li YB, Crook N, Peng B, Niu T. Laparoscopic splenectomy: a surgeon's experience of 302 patients with analysis of postoperative complications. Surg Endosc. 2013;27:3564–71.
22. Cai YQ, Liu XB, Peng B. Should we routinely transfuse platelet for immune thrombocytopenia patients with platelet count less than 10 x 10(9)/L who underwent laparoscopic splenectomy? World J Surg. 2014;38:2267–72.
23. Listed N. National Cancer Institute sponsored study of classifications of non-Hodgkin's lymphomas: summary and description of a working formulation for clinical usage. The Non-Hodgkin's Lymphoma Pathologic Classification Project. Cancer. 1982;49(10):2112–35.
24. Harris NL, Jaffe ES, Stein H, et al. A revised European-American classification of lymphoid neoplasms: a proposal from the International Lymphoma Study Group. Blood. 1994;2(5):1361–92.
25. Riad R, Omar W, Kotb M, et al. Role of PET/CT in malignant pediatric lymphoma. Eur J Nucl Med Mol Imaging. 2010;37(2):319–29.
26. Cheah CY, Hofman MS, Dickinson M, et al. Limited role for surveillance PET–CT scanning in patients with diffuse large B-cell lymphoma in complete metabolic remission following primary therapy. Br J Cancer. 2013;109(2):312–7.
27. Albano D, Patti C, Matranga D, et al. Whole-body diffusion-weighted MR and FDG-PET/CT in Hodgkin Lymphoma: predictive role before treatment and early assessment after two courses of ABVD. Eur J Radiol. 2018;103(6):90–8.
28. Healy NA, Conneely JB, Mahon S, et al. Primary splenic lymphoma presenting with ascites. Rare Tumors. 2011;3(2):e25.
29. Jasminka JR, Igor A. The World Health Organization classification of lymphomas. Croat Med J. 2002;43(5):527–34.
30. Ahmann DL, Kiely JM, Harrison EG, et al. Malignant lymphoma of the spleen. A review of 49 cases in which the diagnosis was made at splenectomy. Cancer. 1966;19(4):461–9.
31. Ke XY. Lymphoma. Beijing: Scientific and Technical Documentation Press; 2009.
32. Kehoe J, Straus DJ. Primary lymphoma of the spleen: clinical features and outcome after splenectomy. Cancer. 2015;62(7):1433–8.
33. Iwakiri Y. Pathophysiology of portal hypertension. Semin Liver Dis. 2014;23(1):6–10.
34. Garcia TG. Portal hypertension. Curr Opin Gastroenterol. 2005;16(3):282–9.
35. Iwakiri Y. Pathophysiology of portal hypertension. Gastroenterol Clin N Am. 1992;21(1):1–14.
36. Kimura K, Ohto M, Matsutani S, et al. Relative frequencies of portosystemic pathways and renal shunt formation through the "posterior" gastric vein: portography study in 460 patients. Hepatology. 1990;12(4):725–8.
37. Ito K, Higuchi M, Kada T, et al. CT of acquired abnormalities of the portal venous system. Radiographics. 1997;17(4):897–917.
38. Taylor CR. Computed tomography in the assessment of the portal venous system. J Clin Gastroenterol. 1992;14(2):167–72.
39. Tang SH, Zeng WZ, Wu XL, et al. Formation of collateral circulation in patients with cirrhotic por-

tal hypertension and its clinical significance. J Clin Hepatol. 2016;32(8):1613–6.
40. Zhao LQ, He W, Ji M, et al. 64-Row multidetector computed tomography portal venography of gastric variceal collateral circulation. World J Gastroenterol. 2010;16(8):1003–7.
41. Reiberger T, Püspök A, Schoder M, et al. Austrian consensus guidelines on the management and treatment of portal hypertension (Billroth III). Wien Klin Wochenschr. 2017;129(3):135–58.
42. Yoshida H, Mamada Y, Taniai N, et al. New trends in surgical treatment for portal hypertension. Hepatol Res. 2010;39(10):1044–51.
43. Wang XY, Xiu DR. Controversy and reflection of surgery for portal hypertension. J Clin Surg. 2018;26(5):325–6.
44. Yin L, Liu H, Zhang Y, et al. The surgical treatment for portal hypertension: a systematic review and meta-analysis. Isrn Gastroenterol. 2013;2013(2):1–10.
45. Gur I, Diggs BS, Orloff SL. Surgical portosystemic shunts in the era of TIPS and liver transplantation are still relevant. HPB. 2014;16(5):481–93.
46. Xin Z, Qingguang L, Yingmin Y. Total laparoscopic versus open splenectomy and esophagogastric devascularization in the management of portal hypertension: a comparative study. Dig Surg. 2009;26(6):499–505.
47. Cai Y, Liu Z, Liu X. Laparoscopic versus open splenectomy for portal hypertension: a systematic review of comparative studies. Surg Innov. 2014;21(4):442–7.
48. Cai YQ, Zhou J, Chen XD, et al. Laparoscopic splenectomy is an effective and safe intervention for hypersplenism secondary to liver cirrhosis. Surg Endosc. 2011;25(12):3791–7.
49. Klein B, Stein M, Kuten A. Splenomegaly and solitary spleen metastasis in solid tumors. Cancer. 1987;60(1):100–6.
50. Kamaya A, Weinstein S, Desser TS. Multiple lesions of the spleen: differential diagnosis of cystic and solid lesions. Semin Ultrasound CT MRI. 2006;27(5):389–403.
51. Wang JH, Ma XL, Ren FY, et al. Multi-modality imaging findings of splenic hamartoma: a report of nine cases and review of the literature. Abdom Imaging. 2013;38(1):154–62.
52. Pang WB, Chen YJ. Diagnosis and management of splenic cysts. Int J Surg. 2008;35(6):407–9.
53. Corcione F, Cuccurullo D, Caiazzo P, et al. Laparoscopic partial splenectomy for a splenic pseudocyst. Surg Endosc. 2003;17(11):1850.
54. Willcox TM, Speer RW, Schlinkert RT, et al. Hemangioma of the spleen: presentation, diagnosis, and management. J Gastrointest Surg. 2000;4(6):611–3.
55. Qin XG, Huang Y, Lin JL, et al. Discussion of surgical indications for splenic hemangioma. Chinese J Clin (Electr Ed). 2013;7(11):5147–8.
56. Zhou YJ, Gu J. Research progress on metastatic carcinoma of the spleen. Chinese J General Surg. 2008;23(2):150–2.
57. Vinnicombe SJ, Reznek RH. Computerised tomography in the staging of Hodgkin's disease and non-Hodgkin's lymphoma. Eur J Nucl Med Mol Imaging. 2003;30(1):42–55.
58. Jiang HC, Qiao HQ. Spleen surgery. Shenyang: Liaoning Science and Technology Publishing House; 2007.
59. Jiang HC, Dai WJ. Classification of splenic injury and choose of surgical procedures. J Clin Surg. 2006;14(7):404–5.
60. Zhang Y, Song JN, Song LX, et al. Laparoscopic splenectomy for traumatic spleen rupture. Chinese J Minim Invas Surg. 2005;5(11):886–7.
61. Jin XB, Wang DQ, Xu XY, et al. Spleen-preserving treatment of traumatic splenic rupture. Zhejiang J Traumat Surg. 2008;13(2):130–1.
62. Yang E, Wu F, Xiao TX, et al. Clinical application of laparoscopic techniques in treatment of traumatic spleen rupture. Chinese J Bases Clin Gen Surg. 2014;21(12):1570–2.
63. Cai YQ, Li CL, Zhang H, et al. Emergency laparoscopic partial splenectomy for ruptured spleen: a case report. World J Gastroenterol. 2014;20(46):17670–3.

4 Perioperative Management of Laparoscopic Splenic Surgery and Application of Enhanced Recovery After Surgery (ERAS)

Yunqiang Cai, Lingwei Meng, Man Zhang, and Bing Peng

4.1 Background

Enhanced recovery after surgery (ERAS) is a new therapeutic concept emerging with the introduction and application of the model of bio-psycho-social medicine. It refers to a series of perioperative optimized treatment measures based on evidence-based medical evidence. Perioperative period refers to the whole process around the surgery, from the time when the patient decides to undergo surgery to the time of basic rehabilitation, including the period before, during, and after the operation. Specifically, it refers to the period from the decision of operative treatment, until the end of the treatment related to the operation, about 5–7 days before the surgery to 7–12 days after the surgery [1]. Along with the treatment of the patients, ERAS requires to reduce the patient's traumatic stress reaction and their complications and to accelerate the patient rehabilitation as much as possible. The concept of ERAS was first proposed by Danish surgeon Kehlet [2] in 1997, and it has been gradually applied to various surgical fields, including gastrointestinal surgery, obstetrics and gynecology, urology, orthopedics, cardiothoracic surgery, and so on [3–6]. Nevertheless, splenic surgery has not been made independent from hepatobiliary and pancreatic surgery, so the application of ERAS in splenic surgery is rarely mentioned separately. On the other hand, since Delaitre et al. [7] completed the world's first laparoscopic splenectomy (LS) in 1991, LS has been increasingly applied in the treatment of various benign and malignant splenic diseases due to the advantages of small trauma, rapid recovery, and short postoperative hospitalization, and its safety and effectiveness have been increasingly recognized [8, 9]. Currently, LS has become the first choice for the treatment of surgical diseases of normal to medium-sized spleen. Therefore, we refer to the existing literature and guidelines and introduce the application of ERAS concept in laparoscopic splenic surgery based on the clinical practice of our center.

4.2 Preoperative Preparations

4.2.1 Strict Identification of the Indications of LS

Laparoscopic splenectomy (LS) has the advantages of less surgery trauma, less general reaction, and quicker postoperative recovery, which is consistent with the concept of ERAS. However, LS is more difficult and risky than open surgery, so the indications of LS must be strictly identified in order to safely carry out the operation

Y. Cai · L. Meng · M. Zhang · B. Peng (✉)
West China Hospital, Sichuan University, Chengdu, China

B. Peng (ed.), *Laparoscopic Surgery of the Spleen*, https://doi.org/10.1007/978-981-16-1216-9_4

and the ERAS. At present, it is considered that the theoretical indications of open abdominal splenectomy are identical with those of LS, but there are still some relative contraindications of LS, such as portal hypertensive pathological spleen, splenomegaly, severe perisplenic inflammation and adhesion, tortuous vessels, and tortuous anatomical structure. In addition to the same contraindications as open splenectomy, absolute contraindications mainly include those with difficulty in tolerating pneumoperitoneum and those with acute massive hemorrhage of traumatic rupture of the spleen complicated with unstable blood circulation. In conclusion, the indications of laparoscopic splenectomy should be identified based on the proficiency and experience of the surgeon. The key is not the disease or the size of the spleen, but the safe completion of the operation without or with few complications [10].

4.2.2 Preoperative Education

Laparoscopic splenectomy is different from traditional surgery, so patients may have different degrees of panic and anxiety before surgery, worrying about whether the laparoscopic surgery could completely remove the diseased part of the spleen, how the treatment effect would be, what the possible risks during surgery are, and whether there is postoperative pain and complications. In addition, the trauma, anesthesia, and the stimulation of the disease itself can cause a series of neuroendocrine reactions, resulting in physiological dysfunction and different degrees of psychological stress of the patients, thus weakening their body's defense and tolerance to the operation and affecting their prognosis. Studies have found that preoperative information about surgery and perioperative treatment can be introduced to patients and their families through oral presentation, text, and multimedia communication, which can not only help reduce patients' tension and anxiety about anesthesia and surgery but also enhance patients' compliance [11]. Due to the particularity of LS, the contents of the information should include:

1. The way of anesthesia and the process of laparoscopic surgery
2. The characteristics of laparoscopic splenic surgery and the possible conversion to open surgery, as well as the explanation to the patient that such conversion does not mean the operation fails
3. The advantages, prognosis, possible perioperative complications, and the corresponding treatment methods
4. The purpose and specific process of ERAS scheme for laparoscopic splenectomy, in order to gain the cooperation of patients and their family members
5. The do's and don'ts after discharge and the key points of postoperative reexamination

4.2.3 Preoperative Nutrition Screening and Nutritional Support Therapy

Most patients with splenic disease are not malnourished preoperatively, but it would occur in patients with portal hypertension associated with hepatic cirrhosis or patients with malignant tumors. Studies have found that preoperative severe malnutrition increases the incidence of postoperative complications, but the existing clinical evidence does not recommend routine preoperative nutritional support in all patients [12]. For patients with a nutritional risk screening score (NRS) 2002 of ≥3 points, preoperative nutritional support is recommended [13]. Oral or enteral nutrition is prioritized in preoperative nutrition support. Only for patients with difficulty in feeding or with enteral malnutrition, parenteral nutrition could be taken into consideration. It is recommended to monitor serum prealbumin to reflect the improvement of the nutritional status of the body [14]. Daily nutrition goals should be set according to the specific physical condition of each patient. According to the guidelines of European Society of Parenteral and Enteral Nutrition (ESPEN), for patients undergoing selective operation, if there is severe malnutrition, (a) weight loss >10% within 6 months; (b) body mass index (BMI) <18.5 kg/m^2; and (c) albumin <30 g/L (no liver or renal dysfunction), it is recommended to consult a specialist for nutritional support therapy [15].

4.2.4 Preoperative Fasting and Water Deprivation

It was previously believed that preoperative fasting for 8–12 h and water deprivation for 4 h could reduce the risk of asphyxiation or aspiration pneumonia due to the vomiting reflex during anesthesia or surgery. However, current clinical practice has shown that prolonged fasting can increase insulin resistance and discomfort after abdominal surgery. Furthermore, guidelines from the European and American anesthesiology societies do not recommend fasting or water deprivation from midnight before surgery. The experience of our center shows that for patients without gastrointestinal motility disturbance, solid food should be fasted 6 h before induction of anesthesia, and liquid food should be fasted 2 h before. Some studies have pointed out that this measure, instead of increasing the risk of gastric retention, can relieve patients' hunger and thirst and reduce patients' anxiety and postoperative insulin resistance [16, 17].

4.2.5 Preoperative Intestinal Preparation

The requirement for intestinal preparation before laparoscopic splenectomy is low, and the evidence of evidence-based medicine (EBM) shows that mechanical intestinal preparation does not reduce the incidence of postoperative complications. Instead, it may lead to dehydration and electrolyte disorder and increase patient discomfort, especially in elderly patients. Our practice suggests that routine mechanical intestinal preparation is not recommended for laparoscopic splenectomy.

4.2.6 Prophylactic Use of Antibiotics

Studies have shown that prophylactic use of antibiotics to achieve effective concentrations in local tissues and correct skin preparation can reduce the risk of surgical site infections (SSIS) [18]. It is recommended that for patients who undergo LS, intravenous administration should be carried out within 30–60 min prior to incision of the skin. If the operation time is longer than 3 h, or longer than twice of the half-life period of the drug, or if intraoperative bleeding is over 1500 mL for adults, a single dose should be added during the operation [19, 20].

4.2.7 Preoperative Nasogastric Tube Indwelling

Meta-analysis has shown that for hepatectomy, the indwelled nasogastric tube can increase postoperative discomfort and stress response of patients, cause or aggravate pulmonary complications, and delay patients' postoperative dietary recovery [21]. Similarly, conventional nasogastric tube decompression is not recommended for LS. Our experience shows that the nasogastric tube is not routinely placed preoperatively. For patients with obvious gastric distension during laparoscopic exploration, the nasogastric tube can be placed to remit gastric pneumatosis and discharge gastric contents in order to obtain a good visual field. However, it should be removed after the operation.

4.2.8 Prophylactic Antithrombotic Therapy

After splenectomy, platelets increase temporarily or continuously in most patients, which may lead to an increase in the occurrence of venous thrombosis. For patients undergoing laparoscopic splenectomy, prophylactic antithrombotic therapy is performed according to the perioperative standard of prophylactic anti-thrombotic therapy for laparoscopic pancreatic surgery in our center [22].

4.3 Intraoperative Measures

4.3.1 Incision Selection

The placement of trocars in laparoscopic splenectomy varies among different centers. Our center routinely adopts the method of 4-trocar splenectomy. After the splenectomy, the spleen is put into a specimen bag and cut into pieces. For patients with malignant tumors or those who need to retain intact spleen for pathological diagnosis, specimens should be removed through extended incision. Most of the specimens are taken out through extended navel incision in our center, and suprapubic transverse incision is also selected in some centers.

4.3.2 Prevention of Intraoperative Hypothermia

Studies have found that hypothermia significantly increases the occurrence of bleeding and blood transfusion [23], while patients who maintain normal body temperature intraoperatively have a lower incidence of postoperative cardiac complications [24]. The standard "dry-cold" CO_2 gas (temperature 20–21 °C/68–70 °F, humidity 0.0002%) used in laparoscopic surgery can lead to hypothermia [25]. Therefore, in laparoscopic splenectomy, multiple methods should be used to prevent the occurrence of hypothermia, for example, operating room temperature should not be too low, and the usage of liquid heating device, heater, peritoneal washing after warmed, and other measures can be carried out to maintain the patient's intraoperative core body temperature above 36 °C (or 97 °F).

4.3.3 Placement of Intraoperative Abdominal Drainage Tube

There is still a lack of sufficient evidence to support the routine placement of abdominal drainage tubes after splenectomy. The placement of drainage tube in laparoscopic splenectomy depends on the intraoperative specific circumstances and is recommended for patients with severe anatomical adhesions, larger area wounded, and more risks of bleeding and pancreatic leakage (if pancreatectomy is combined).

4.4 Postoperative Measures

4.4.1 Early Postoperative Oral Feeding and Nutritional Support

Postoperative nutritional support is closely related to healing, especially for malnourished patients. Postoperative oral feeding should be resumed as soon as possible. Most patients with LS begin to orally drink clear water on postoperative day 1 (POD 1) and then orally take liquid or semi-liquid diet, and those who are tolerant can gradually transit to normal diets [26]. Routine enteral or parenteral nutrition support is not recommended for patients after LS. Instead, enteral and parenteral nutrition support is only used in patients who cannot orally take for a long time due to various reasons or in patients with malnutrition. And the nutrition scheme is made according to the individual situation of patients [27].

4.4.2 Prevention and Treatment of Postoperative Nausea and Vomiting

Postoperative nausea and vomiting are common adverse reactions. Severe nausea and vomiting may lead to electrolyte loss and internal environment disturbance and delay the oral intake, causing negative impacts on the prognosis of patients. Thus, for the high-risk patients with the occurrence of postoperative nausea and vomiting (PONV), it is recommended to preventatively combine a variety of drugs [28]. For the patients with two of the following risk factors, (a) female, (b) non-smoker, (c) history of motion sickness or PONV, and (d) postoperative opioid use, it is recommended to administrate dexamethasone when induction of anesthesia or to administrate 5-hydroxytryptamlne receptor (5-HR) antagonist at the end of surgery. For patients with three of the above factors, general anesthesia with propofol and remifentanil is recommended rather than inhaled anesthesia, dexamethasone should be given during the induction of anesthesia, and before the end of the surgery, 5-HR antagonist should be administrated. The use of a 5-HR antagonist is recommended for PONV treatment [29].

4.4.3 Postoperative Analgesia Management

Postoperative pain is a series of physiological, psychological, and behavioral reactions that occur after the body is stimulated by surgery. It affects patients' early postoperative activity and gastrointestinal functional recovery and increases anxiety, leading to much more occurrences of venous thromboembolism, prolonged hospitalization, and higher rehospitalization rate. Therefore, pain management is a fairly important issue in ERAS. As a minimally invasive surgery, laparoscopy significantly alleviates postoperative pain in patients compared with larger incision in open surgery. However, with the improvement of people's living standard and the deepening of pain awareness, it is the patients' right to request painlessness. Analgesia options include intravenous controlled analgesia, incision infiltration analgesia, drug analgesia, psychological comfort, and so on [30]. The choice of analgesic drugs should be individualized. According to our experience, before the end of the operation, laparoscopic trocar hole is used for incision infiltration anesthesia with long-acting local anesthetics. Ropivacaine and bupivacaine are firstly recommended. For postoperative pain, oral intake of non-selective nonsteroidal anti-inflammatory drugs (NSAIDs) or selective cyclooxygenase-2 (COX-2) inhibitors can be selected, and opioid analgesics can be applied for severe pain.

4.4.4 Early Postoperative Activities

Early postoperative activities play a very important role in postoperative functional recovery, which can not only promote the recovery of muscle, respiratory system, and gastrointestinal function but also reduce the occurrence of postoperative thromboembolism and insulin resistance [31]. Besides, active out-of-bed activities can make the removal of catheter earlier and reduce the probability of postoperative urinary tract infection. Patients with laparoscopic surgery are advised to exercise on the first day after surgery. A reasonable and clear plan should be made to guide patients to exercise in the early postoperative period, and the implementation of the plan should be recorded and supervised [4, 28].

4.4.5 Postoperative Removal of Abdominal Drainage Tube

In our center, a drainage tube is routinely placed after LS for the monitoring of pancreatic leakage, bleeding, and drainage of seroperitoneum. If the abdominal drainage fluid is less than 10 mL or none on POD 1, the abdominal drainage tube can be extracted immediately after the splenic fossa hydrops is excluded by color ultrasound or CT imaging. If the drainage fluid is more than 10 mL, the drainage fluid amylase should be measured on POD 3 to confirm that no pancreatic fistula has occurred. If there is no pancreatic fistula and no special symptoms (fever, left upper abdominal distension, abdominal pain, etc.) observed, the abdominal drainage tube could be removed. During the indwelling of the abdominal drainage tube, attention should be paid to ensuring its patency, as unsmooth drainage of the seroperitoneum may lead to effusion or secondary infection or even the formation of abdominal abscess.

4.4.6 Postoperative Catheter Removal Timing

Catheters are routinely placed intraoperatively in our center, and prolonged catheter indwelling after surgery will increase the risk of urinary tract infection. Evidence-based medicine recommends the use of transurethral indwelling catheterization and early removal after surgery. Usually we extract catheters on POD 1. But for patients with symptomatic benign prostatic hyperplasia (BPH) (especially in elderly patients), tamsulosin hydrochloride sustained release capsules can be administrated after admission to hospital, and finasteride can be combined when necessary, until POD 3 when catheters are extracted. Generally, patients can urinate smoothly, and the relocation of catheters after pulling it out early can be avoided to reduce the risk of urinary tract infection.

4.4.7 Reduction of Postoperative SRMD

Reducing surgical stress is the core concept of ERAS. Stress-related mucosal disease (SRMD) is a vital manifestation of acute gastrointestinal dysfunction caused by severe stress, especially after major surgeries. Prevention and treatment of SRMD will improve perioperative safety and shorten hospital stay. Current studies have confirmed that proton pump inhibitors can effectively prevent SRMD and reduce the risk of postoperative upper gastrointestinal bleeding and death [31].

4.5 Discharge Criteria

According to the discharge criteria for laparoscopic distal pancreatectomy [28], our center believes that patients who meet the following criteria can be discharged:

1. No signs of infection such as fever, abdominal pain, or increased blood count
2. Tolerant of orally intaking solid food
3. Self-defecation
4. Able to reach a certain level of activity (out-of-bed activity for more than 4 h/day)
5. Good healing of incisions

4.6 Conclusions and Future Prospects

The implementation of ERAS concept aims to reduce perioperative stress response of patients, accelerate postoperative rehabilitation, shorten hospitalization time, and save social resources while treating diseases. The advantages of LS are less trauma, rapid recovery, and short hospitalization, which is consistent with the concept of ERAS. However, when applying ERAS concept to laparoscopic splenectomy, it is necessary to comprehensively consider the complexity of splenic surgery and the characteristics of laparoscopic surgery, so as to formulate ERAS scheme suitable for LS. With the development of the clinical practice of laparoscopic spleen surgery and its further integration with the idea of ERAS, we believe that formulation of the standard and guidance could be promoted. It should be noted that, in the clinical practice of the ERAS, we have to take the characteristics of the medical institute and actual situation into full consideration, to optimize measures and to make an individualized ERAS scheme for different patients.

References

1. Bao SM. Perioperative holistic nursing care of patients. Chin Nutr HC. 2013;23(8):4215.
2. Kehlet H. Multimodal approach to control postoperative pathophysiology and rehabilitation. Br J Anaesth. 1997;78(5):606–17.
3. Mortensen K, Nilsson M, Slim K, et al. Consensus guidelines for enhanced recovery after gastrectomy Enhanced Recovery After Surgery (ERAS®) Society recommendations. Br J Surg. 2014;101(10):1209–29.
4. Lassen K, Coolsen MME, Slim K, et al. Guidelines for perioperative care for pancreaticoduodenectomy: Enhanced Recovery After Surgery (ERAS®) Society recommendations. Clin Nutr. 2012;31(6):817–30.
5. Gustafsson UO, Scott MJ, Schwenk W, et al. Guidelines for perioperative care in elective colonic surgery: Enhanced Recovery After Surgery (ERAS®) Society recommendations. Clin Nutr. 2012;31(6):783–800.
6. Nygren J, Thacker J, Carli F, et al. Guidelines for perioperative care in elective rectal/pelvic surgery: Enhanced Recovery After Surgery (ERAS®) Society recommendations. Clin Nutr. 2012;31(6):801–16.
7. Delaitre B, Maignien B. Splenectomy by the laparoscopic approach: report of a case. Presse Med. 1991;20(44):2263.
8. Wu JM, Lai IR, Yuan RH, et al. Laparoscopic splenectomy for idiopathic thrombocytopenic purpura. Am J Surg. 2004;187(6):720–3.
9. Knauer EM, Ailawadi G, Yahanda A, et al. 101 laparoscopic splenectomies for the treatment of benign and malignant hematologic disorders. Am J Surg. 2003;186(5):500–4.
10. Bhandarkar DS, Katara AN, Mittal G, et al. Prevention and management of complications of laparoscopic splenectomy. Indian J Surg. 2011;73(5):324–30.
11. Aarts M, Okrainec A, Glicksman A, et al. Adoption of enhanced recovery after surgery (ERAS) strategies for colorectal surgery at academic teaching hospitals and impact on total length of hospital stay. Surg Endosc. 2012;26(2):442–50.
12. Probst P, Haller S, Dorr-Harim C, et al. Nutritional risk in major abdominal surgery: protocol of a prospective observational trial to assess the prognostic value of different nutritional scores in pancreatic surgery. JMIR Res Protoc. 2015;4(4):132.
13. Bozzetti F, Mariani L. Perioperative nutritional support of patients undergoing pancreatic surgery in the age of ERAS. Nutrition. 2014;30(11-12):1267–71.
14. van Stijn MF, Korkic-Halilovic I, Bakker MS, et al. Preoperative nutrition status and postoperative outcome in elderly general surgery patients: a systematic review. JPEN J Parenter Enteral Nutr. 2013;37(1):37–43.
15. Schindler K, Pernicka E, Laviano A, et al. How nutritional risk is assessed and managed in European hospitals: A survey of 21,007 patients findings from the 2007-2008 cross-sectional nutrition Day survey. Clin Nutr. 2010;29(5):552–9.
16. Committee ASOA. Practice guidelines for preoperative fasting and the use of pharmacologic agents to reduce the risk of pulmonary aspiration: application to healthy patients undergoing elective procedures: an updated report by the American Society of Anesthesiologists Committee on Standards and Practice Parameters. Anesthesiology. 2011;114(3):495.
17. Smith I, Kranke P, Murat I, et al. Perioperative fasting in adults and children: guidelines from the European Society of Anaesthesiology. Eur J Anaesthesiol. 2011;28(8):556–69.
18. Bratzler DW, Houck PM, Workgroup SIPGW. Antimicrobial prophylaxis for surgery: an advisory statement from the National Surgical Infection Prevention Project. Am J Surg. 2005;189(4):395–404.
19. Yang F. Interpretation of guidelines for the clinical application of antimicrobial drugs (2015). Chin J Clin. 2016;9(5):390–3.
20. Revision Working Group of Guidelines for the Clinical Application of Antimicrobial Drugs. Guidelines for The Clinical Application of Antimicrobial Drugs (2015). Beijing: People's Medical Publish House; 2015.
21. Pessaux P, Regimbeau JM, Dondero F, et al. Randomized clinical trial evaluating the need for routine nasogastric decompression after elective hepatic resection. Br J Surg. 2007;94(3):297–303.
22. Zeng Y, Peng B. Laparoscopic pancreatic surgery (1st ed.). Beijing: People's Medical Publishing House; 2017. p. 13–4.
23. Kurz A, Sessler DI, Lenhardt R. Perioperative normothermia to reduce the incidence of surgical-wound infection and shorten hospitalization. N Engl J Med. 1996;334(19):1209–15.
24. Frank SM, Fleisher LA, Breslow MJ, et al. Perioperative maintenance of normothermia reduces the incidence of morbid cardiac events—a randomized clinical trial. JAMA. 1997;277(14):1127–34.
25. Liu LX, Chen YJ, Cang MH, et al. Chinese expert concensus of ERAS of laparoscopic hepatectomy (2017). Chin J Prac Surg. 2017;37(05):517–24.
26. Yamazaki S, Takayama T, Higaki T, et al. Pancrelipase with branched-chain amino acids for preventing nonalcoholic fatty liver disease after pancreaticoduodenectomy. J Gastroenterol. 2016;51(1):55–62.
27. Lidder PG, Lewis S, Duxbury M. Systematic review of postdischarge oral nutritional supplementation in patients undergoing GI surgery. Nutr Clin Pract. 2009;24(3):388–94.
28. Bruns H, Rahbari NN, Löffler T, et al. Perioperative management in distal pancreatectomy: results of a survey in 23 European participating centres of the DISPACT trial and a review of literature. Trials. 2009;10(1):1–12.

29. Carlisle JB. Drugs for preventing postoperative nausea and vomiting: prevention in context. BMJ. 2006;333(7565):448.
30. Leng XS, Jai WD, Miao Y. Expert consensus of general surgery perioperative pain managemen. Chin J GenSurg. 2015;30(2):166–73.
31. Alhazzani W, Alenezi F, Jaeschke RZ, et al. Proton pump inhibitors versus histamine 2 receptor antagonists for stress ulcer prophylaxis in critically ill patients: a systematic review and meta-analysis. Crit Care Med. 2013;41(3):693–705.

5 Laparoscopic Splenectomy (LS)

Lingwei Meng, Sirui Chen, Bo Liao, Chunlin Li, and Bing Peng

5.1 Background

Laparoscopic splenic surgery began in 1991, when Delaitre et al. [1] finished the world's first laparoscopic splenectomy (LS). Initially, LS was mainly used in patients with normal spleen or mild splenomegaly, and it has been currently applied to a variety of diseases leading to splenomegaly [2] and splenic benign and malignant tumors [3, 4]. Compared with open splenectomy (OS), LS has merits of less trauma and pain, with proved effect [5]. It has currently become the standard operation for the treatment of most splenic-related blood diseases [6].

L. Meng · B. Peng (✉)
West China Hospital, Sichuan University, Chengdu, China

S. Chen
Mianyang Center Hospital, Mianyang, China

B. Liao
AVIC 363 Hospital, Chengdu, China

C. Li
Cinical Medical College & Affiliated Hospital of Chengdu University, Chengdu, China

5.2 Indications and Contraindications

5.2.1 Indications

1. Splenic rupture: traumatic, spontaneous, and surgically induced rupture of the spleen
2. Hypersplenism: primary hypersplenism, congestive hypersplenism, and others requiring splenectomy (e.g., (a) significant hypersplenism inducing compression symptoms; (b) severe anemia, especially complicated with hemolytic anemia; (c) considerable degree of thrombocytopenia and bleeding symptoms; (d) granulocytopenia with a history of recurrent infection)
3. Splenic diseases: splenic cyst, benign and malignant splenic tumors, splenic abscess and splenic tuberculosis, wandering spleen, etc.
4. Hematological system diseases: immune thrombocytopenia purpura (ITP), hereditary spherocytosis (complicated with anemia, splenomegaly, hemoglobin less than 100 g/L), hemolytic anemia, β-thalassemia, thrombotic thrombocytopenic purpura, etc.
5. Collateral splenectomy: total or distal pancreatectomy, gastrectomy, colectomy, retroperitoneal mass resection, and other operations requiring collateral splenectomy

B. Peng (ed.), *Laparoscopic Surgery of the Spleen*, https://doi.org/10.1007/978-981-16-1216-9_5

5.2.2 Contradictions

Including relative and absolute contradictions as follows:

5.2.2.1 Absolute Contradictions

1. Patients with poor coagulation function that is difficult to correct or intolerance of operation
2. Patients with poor cardiopulmonary function or intolerance of pneumoperitoneum
3. Patients with poor physical conditions, including poor liver function, who cannot tolerate general anesthesia or surgery

5.2.2.2 Relative Contraindications

1. Patients with splenomegaly (megalosplenia, a spleen with a longitudinal length of >20 cm or a weight of >1000 g; massive-splenomegaly, a spleen with a longitudinal length of >22 cm or a weight of >1200 g), leading to a narrow operating space
2. Patients with previous upper abdominal surgical history, whose abdominal adhesions might be serious and whose spleen is not easily exposed

5.3 Preoperative Assessment and Preparation

Preoperative enhanced abdominal CT is routinely performed in our center to determine the volume of the spleen and to assess the relationship between the spleen and surrounding tissues.

Routine preoperative examinations can be taken into consideration according to the patients' condition, including blood cell counts, coagulation function, blood type, liver and kidney function, electrolyte, infectious disease screening (hepatitis B, C, HIV/AIDS, and syphilis), and electrocardiogram examination. Echocardiography and pulmonary function test (applicable for the elderly or those of related past medical history). Antibiotics should be administered within 30–60 min before incising the skin. If the operation time is longer than 3 h, or longer than the half-value period of the drug, or if intraoperative bleeding is over 1500 mL for adults, a single dose should be added during the operation [7].

The above principles are applicable no matter for emergency or elective laparoscopic splenectomy. However, there are some special considerations for elective surgery for patients with special diseases, which are listed as follows:

For patients with hematological system disease, abdominal B-mode ultrasound examination should be performed to ascertain whether there are gallstones.

For elderly patients or patients with liver cirrhosis, operation risk should be fully assessed. Attention should be paid to improving the patient's systemic conditions, blood coagulation function, hypoalbuminemia, and anemia. Special care should be taken to hematology relevant examination, hepatic and renal function. We can also check about the degree of varix on gastric fundus by gastroscopy. Adequate preoperative assessment and preparation should be done to minimize perioperative risk.

For patients with ITP, preoperative hormone impulse therapy (dexamethasone 10 mg/day for 3 consecutive days) and intraoperative administration of hormone (dexamethasone 10 mg/day) are routinely carried out. Postoperative adjustment of hormone dosage should be done in accordance with the patient's platelet recovery. During the treatment of ITP, we made further study on the patients with extremely low platelets (PLT, $<10 \times 10^9$/L) and concluded that for the patients with extremely low PLT, if the coagulation function is normal, preoperative platelet transfusion could be performed irregularly [8–10]. For patients requiring infusion of platelets, infusion should be given after dissection of splenic pedicle intraoperatively.

No matter what kind of disease is involved in laparoscopic splenectomy, the patient and/or his/her family members should be thoroughly informed about the risks of the operation and the possible complications and even the life-threatening situation of the patient. For surgeons, good preoperative communication with patients and/or their family members is a prerequisite for medical safety.

5.4 Surgical Procedures

5.4.1 Surgical Position and Surgeon Position

Surgical position: After the success of general anesthesia, place the patient in the supine anti-Trendelenburg position for about 30° (place head higher than foot horizontally), and pad the left shoulder-back for 15–30°.

Surgeon position and device placement: The surgeon and the laparoscopy navigator are on the right side of the patient, the first assistant is on the left side of the patient, and each of the left and right sides of the patient's head is placed with one monitor, respectively (Fig. 5.1).

5.4.2 Main Steps

5.4.2.1 Pneumoperitoneum Establishment

Usually we place four trocars in LS (Fig. 5.1). First, incise the skin 0.2–0.5 cm above or below the umbilicus, then place Veress needle, connect it to CO_2 pump, and maintain the pneumoperitoneal pressure to 12–14 mmHg. Then place a 10 mm trocar as a 30° laparoscopic observation hole, place a 5 mm trocar at the lower left side of the xiphoid as a vice operation hole of the operator, place a 12 mm trocar at 3 cm below the body surface projection of lower pole of the spleen on the left midclavicular line as a main operation hole, and place a 5 mm trocar below the main operation hole horizontally on the left anterior axillary line as the first assistant operation hole. For the patients with splenomegaly, the main operation hole is located 2 cm below the lower pole of the spleen, and the first assistant operating hole is located on the left anterior axillary line below the level of the lower pole. The position and order of the holes can be adjusted according to the size of the spleen.

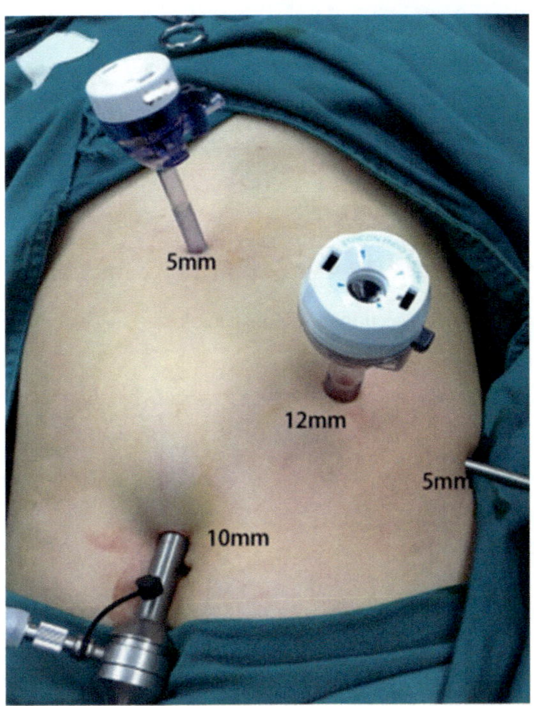

Fig. 5.1 Distribution of trocars

5.4.2.2 Abdominal Cavity Exploration

When exploring the abdominal tissue, pay special attention to the spleen and peri-splenic conditions. For the patient with hematological system disease, special attention should also be paid to the search for the accessory spleen. The exploration should be made carefully, orderly, and gently, to prevent damage to nearby tissue and organ lesions.

5.4.2.3 Dissociation of the Spleen

Open and dissect the splenogastric ligament (Fig. 5.2), splenophrenic ligament (Fig. 5.3), splenocolic ligament (Fig. 5.4), and splenorenal

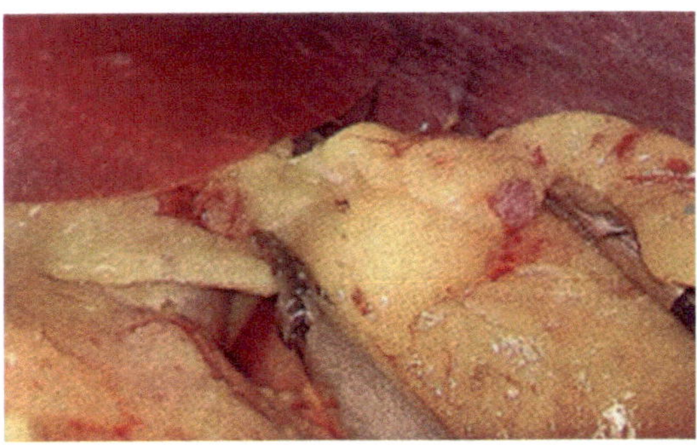

Fig. 5.2 Dissection of splenogastric ligament

ligament (Fig. 5.5) successively with the ultrasonic scalpel or LigaSure. When dissecting the splenogastric ligament near the diaphragm, pay special attention to some of the larger short gastric vessels and do not clamp them directly with the ultrasonic scalpel or LigaSure. Instead, they should be clamped with Hem-o-lok on the basis of full dissociation.

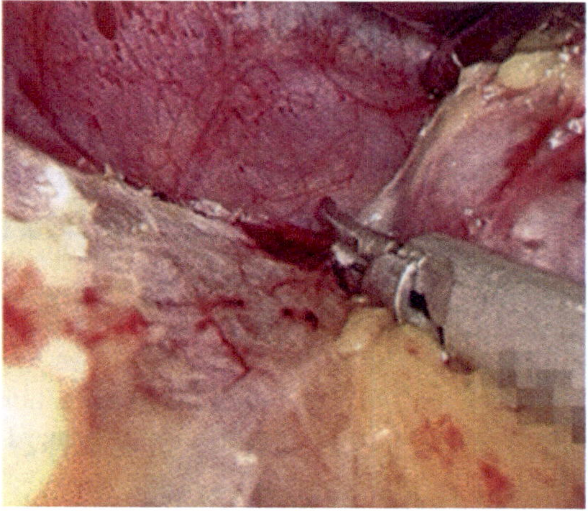

Fig. 5.3 Dissection of diaphragmatic ligament

5.4.2.4 Exposure and Dissection of the Splenic Pedicle

Usually the dissection of primary branch of splenic pedicle is performed. After the spleen is completely dissociated, expose the splenic pedicle, and dissect the splenic pedicle with an endoscopic linear cutting stapler (Fig. 5.6) to completely stop the bleeding.

5.4.2.5 Extraction of the Spleen

Put the spleen into a special specimen bag (Fig. 5.7), crush it with grasping forceps, and take it out.

5.4.2.6 Placement of the Drainage Tube

Observe if there is bleeding from the splenic pedicle and fossa (Fig. 5.8). Then place hemostatic materials, and place an orthopedic drainage tube in the splenic fossa (Fig. 5.9) to monitor if there

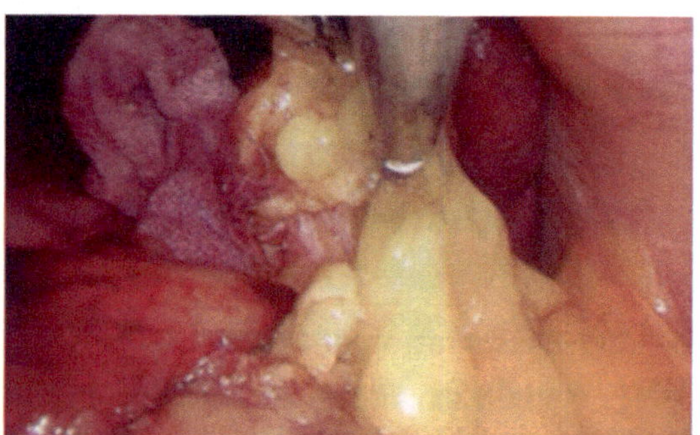

Fig. 5.4 Dissection of splenocolic ligament

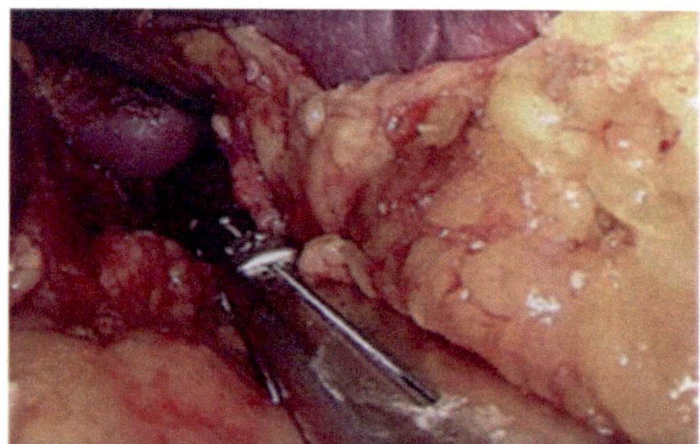

Fig. 5.6 Dissection of splenic pedicle

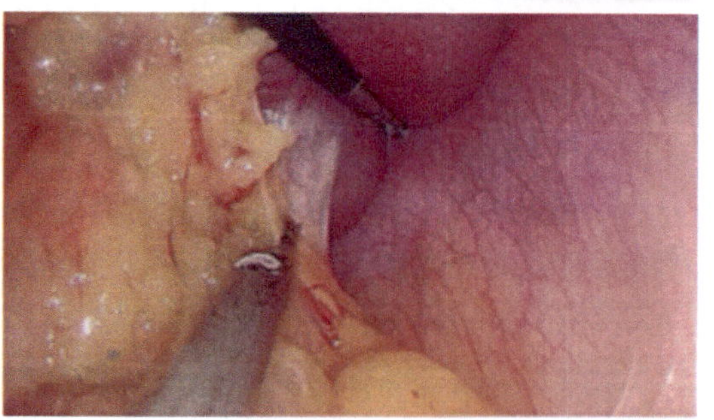

Fig. 5.5 Dissection of splenorenal ligament

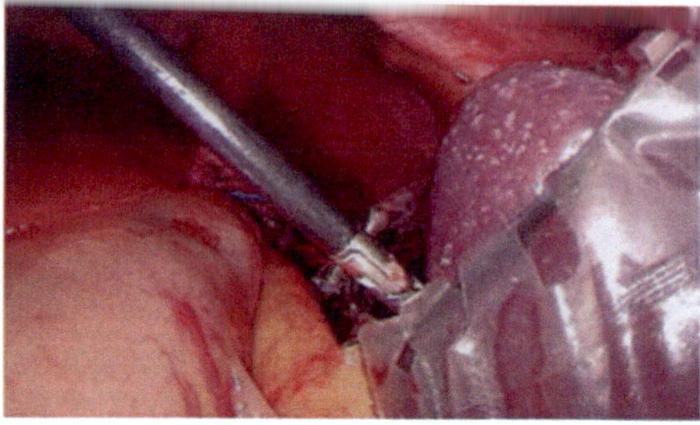

Fig. 5.7 Extraction of the spleen

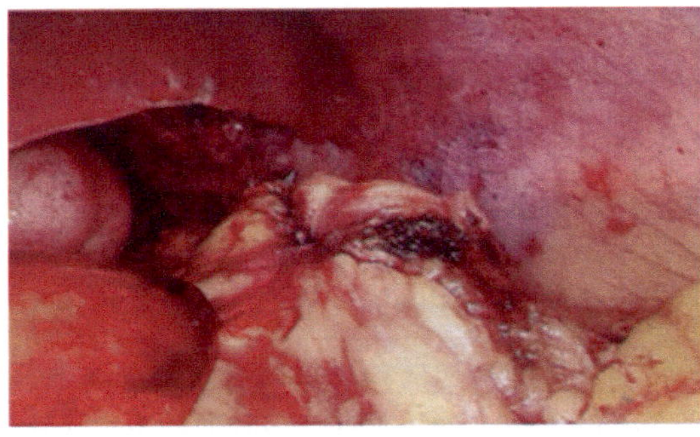

Fig. 5.8 Observation of bleeding from the splenic pedicle and fossa (the picture above shows no bleeding from the broken end of the splenic pedicle)

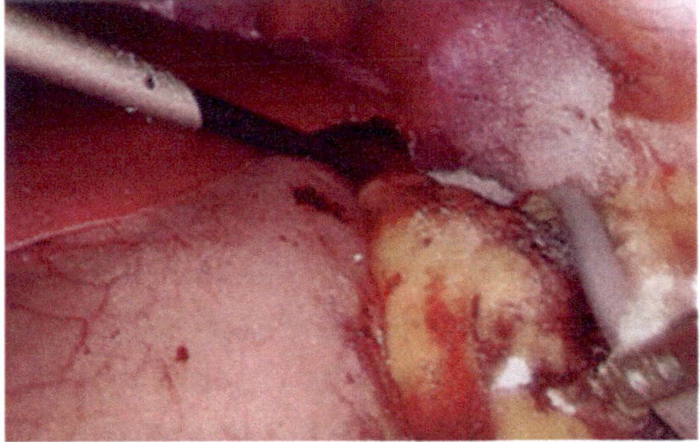

Fig. 5.9 Placement of an orthopedic drainage tube

is bleeding from the broken end of the splenic pedicle or pancreatic fistula postoperatively and simultaneously prevent the accumulation of peritoneal exudate.

5.4.2.7 Quit the Pneumoperitoneum and Suture the Incision

5.5 Key Surgical Techniques

5.5.1 Choice of Approach

Generally, the "upper pole" approach is adopted to open the splenogastric ligaments and dissect them from bottom to top. Intraoperatively, careful operation should be performed to avoid damaging the spleen and other nearby organs or blood vessels.

5.5.2 Dissociation of Superior Splenic Pole

Since the superior splenic pole is adjacent to the stomach and the diaphragm where short gastric vessels are located inside, leading to difficult exposure and narrow operating space, improper handling may cause bleeding and the stomach and diaphragm injury. Therefore, during the operation process, we must pay attention to protecting the short gastric vessels, especially in patients with splenomegaly or obesity. Bear in mind that we should try not to use ultrasonic scalpel or LigaSure to coagulate and close short gastric vessels directly. Instead, clamp it with Hem-o-lok after clearly identifying its contour and its adjacent tissues in order to ensure safety. If it is accidently hurt, massive intraoperative bleeding would be caused, which will not only affect the vision but also make it vulnerable to convert to open surgery for novices, losing the significance of minimally invasive surgery. Thus, special attention should be paid.

5.5.3 Do's and Don'ts When Dissecting Peri-splenic Ligaments

If the diameter of the vessels is larger than 3 mm, they should be ligated with thread or Hem-o-lok clipping as much as possible, instead of ultrasonic scalpel, which should not be used directly if possible. Owing to the fluctuation of postoperative blood pressure, the clipped vessels would be reopened, leading to postoperative hemorrhage, and even requiring secondary surgical treatment. Studies have pointed out [11] that it is safe and reliable to clip blood vessels directly with the ultrasonic scalpel if their diameters are smaller than 2–3 mm, and the bipolar electrocoagulation system may be safe and reliable for blood vessels whose diameter is smaller than 7 mm. In addition, the endoscopic plastic composite clip or titanium clip is safe and reliable for almost all the blood vessels that can be clipped. In general, vessels with the diameter less than 3 mm are directly handled with the ultrasonic scalpel or LigaSure in general, and larger vessels with the diameter larger than 3 mm are clipped with silk thread or Hem-o-lok or titanium clip of different sizes in our center. These operations have been proven to be safe in clinical practice.

5.5.4 Notices for Assistants

During the operation, all the operations of the assistant should be carried out within the field of vision, so as to prevent the injury of adjacent tissues or organs such as the stomach, colon, spleen, and liver during the exposure, causing unnecessary damage to the patient.

5.5.5 Trocar Placement and Precautions

The trocar at the bellybutton should be oriented toward the spleen to reduce the distortion of the observation hole. The placement of trocars should be in full consideration of the size of the spleen; especially for patients with splenomegaly, trocar should be arranged according to the specific conditions.

5.5.6 Abdominal Exploration

Before splenectomy, a thorough abdominal exploration should be carried out to check whether there is an accessory spleen. If the accessory spleen remains in the abdominal cavity, the therapeutic effect of hematological system diseases or malignant tumors will be significantly affected.

5.6 Special Intraoperative Circumstances and Handling Skills

5.6.1 Handling Skills for Severe Abdominal Adhesions

For partial abdominal adhesions, especially for patients with a history of splenic embolism, peri-splenic adhesions are especially serious. In this circumstance, be patient when dissecting the peri-splenic tissues, and find the correct interstitial space because hemorrhage caused by splenic lesion is hard to control. If it is difficult to complete peri-splenic dissociation, dissect the splenic pedicle before its dissociation so as to reduce the risk of bleeding. Dissociating adhesions should be carried out close to the spleen to prevent damage to the adjacent tissues or organs such as the stomach and colon.

5.6.2 Handling Skills for Splenic Pedicle

For handling the splenic pedicle, it must be clearly exposed to ensure that the dissociation of the spleen is complete, the splenic pedicle is thin enough, and the pancreatic tail and splenic pedicle tissues are carefully separated, so as to reduce the injury of pancreas and the risk of the occurrence of pancreatic fistula. The size of Endo-GIA should be selected according to the thickness of splenic pedicle, for example, the white one (1.0 mm thickness) is mostly selected in our center. And it would be better to wait for a 30-s squeezing after clip before triggering. Owing to the possibility of failure of Endo-GIA to successfully clamp and cut the major vessels, massive bleeding may occur, requiring blood transfusion or even conversion to open surgery. Therefore, after the operation, special attention should be paid to checking whether there is bleeding in the spleen pedicle, fossa, etc. If there is bleeding from the spleen pedicle, it can be strengthened by endoscopic suture or by Hem-o-lok clip. If there is no bleeding, conventional suture is not recommended, because there is no medical evidence to prove that this measure can reduce postoperative bleeding or postoperative pancreatic fistula.

5.6.3 Autotransfusion

For patients with non-neoplastic and non-autoimmune diseases, patients with splenomegaly can be considered for autotransfusion of splenic blood. This technique reduces the possibility of postoperative blood transfusion, and there is no external infection or rejection reaction, so it is safer than allogeneic blood transfusion. However, strict aseptic operation must be ensured during the whole process of autotransfusion.

5.6.4 Conversion to Open Surgery

It may happen mainly due to intra-abdominal hemorrhage, which occurs because of the lesion of spleen parenchyma caused by improper operation of the operator or assistant, the splenic rupture caused by accidental injury from the trocar when entering the abdominal cavity, the improper use of Endo-GIA when ligating splenic pedicle, and the hemorrhage due to overly thick splenic pedicle tissues leading to the insufficient clamping. Once the intra-abdominal bleeding is found, compressing to stop bleeding should be carried out without hesitation, rather than blindly electrocoagulation or clamping hemostasis with the ultrasonic scalpel. After using the aspirator to clear the vision, the causes of bleeding should be dealt with respectively. When it is difficult to stop bleeding under the endoscope or too risky to handle with, conversion to open surgery should be immediately carried out. It is vital to remember that converting to open surgery does not mean the operation fails. All the operations should be performed by putting the patient's life first.

5.6.5 Handling Skills for Splenomegaly

For patients with splenomegaly, the main operational difficulty is the narrow vision and limited operating space. Based on our experience, allow the patients to take the right half supine position, pad the left shoulder-back about 60°, and tilt the operating table as anti-Trendelenburg position, which can allow a better exposure and anatomy of the splenic hilus, facilitating the anatomy of inferior pole of spleen and splenorenal ligament and thus the vascular control [2]. In addition, for the handling of patients with splenomegaly, the placement of trocar mainly depends on preoperative detailed physical examination and CT examination. 4-Trocar method is routinely carried out in our center (as mentioned above), and especially, the main operation hole should be located below the horizon of inferior splenic pole, so that we can better dissociate the inferior pole and dissect splenic pedicle from bottom to top with Endo-GIA. For such patients, due to the limited operation space, some of them suffer from significant peri-splenic vascular varix, and it is very important to control the intraoperative hemorrhage. According to our experience, after opening the splenogastric ligament, we find trunk of spleen artery from the upper margin of pancreas, dissociate and ligate the trunk, and perform autotransfusion from the spleen and then dissociate peri-splenic ligaments and dissect vessels in splenic pedicle, so as to reduce the occurrence of intraoperative bleeding risk. For the treatment of short gastric vessels prone to bleeding, first open the posterior parietal peritoneum of the lesser omentum, then fully dissect the back tissue of the short gastric vessels, and clamp the two ends of the vessels, so as to avoid the occurrence of vascular collateral damage and massive bleeding caused by the aimless clamp. At the same time, the thick blood vessels should be ligated with silk thread or with Hem-o-lok clamp in the process of dissociating the spleen. Care should be taken in the process of dissection so as to avoid the rupture of the capsule of the spleen and the difficulty in hemostasis resulting in massive bleeding and the conversion to open surgery. After the operation, the spleen should be put into a specimen bag to avoid leaving any spleen tissue in the abdominal cavity. After the spleen is removed, the abdominal cavity can be flushed with normal saline.

5.7 Postoperative Management and Prevention and Treatment of Complications

5.7.1 Key Points of Postoperative Management

Check the blood routine, liver and renal function, electrolyte, blood amylase, and lipase and remove the gastric tube and the catheter (except for patients with high risk of urinary retention) on postoperative day 1 (POD 1). Observe the gastrointestinal functional recovery, and instruct the postoperative diet and early activities. Observe if there is abdominal drainage fluid and record the volume if any; if less than 10 mL, the abdominal drainage tube can be removed early according to the patient's condition (e.g., no fever, abdominal distension, abdominal pain).

On POD 3, regularly check blood amylase, lipase, drainage fluid amylase, and lipase (if abdominal drainage tube is not removed, which is mainly used to detect the presence of pancreatic fistula and its level), and decide whether to pull out abdominal plasma drainage tube according to the quality and drainage amount of fluid [12]. For patients with postoperative infection, antibiotics should be administrated according to the patient's postoperative body temperature, white blood cell counts, and so on. The antacids, glucocorticoids, and somatostatin should be used in accordance with the patient's conditions.

5.7.2 Prevention and Treatment of Postoperative Complications

5.7.2.1 Complications After Splenectomy

1. Postoperative bleeding: Intra-abdominal bleeding generally occurs within 24–48 h after the surgery [13]. Generally, bleeding from the splenic pedicle is quite dangerous, but rarely seen clinically. When the splenic pedicle is dissected with an Endo-GIA, the integrity of the splenic pedicle should be ensured. Wound surface and splenic bed hemorrhage mainly occurs in patients with severe abdominal adhesion or cirrhosis complicated with portal hypertension. Accurate hemostasis is an effective preventive measure during the operation. The parietal peritoneum of the operation hole must be closed, especially in patients with portal hypertension. Once diagnosed with active intra-abdominal hemorrhage, the patient shall be given the emergency abdominal operational exploration immediately.
2. Pancreatic injury and pancreatic fistula [14]: Pancreas is a common site of injury during splenectomy. Chand et al. [15] reported that such occurrence is 15%, which can be manifested as simple increase of pancreatic enzyme in drainage fluid, peripancreatic effusion, pancreatic abscess, etc. On the one hand, it is associated with unsatisfactory surgical field exposure (such as splenomegaly, severe peri-splenic adhesion); on the other hand, it is related to the close position relationship between the distal pancreas and the splenic hilum. Sometimes, in order to reduce the risk of bleeding when dissection, a part of the pancreatic tissue will be removed with an Endo-GIA. Some scholars also believe that there is a certain correlation between the incidence of pancreatic lesion and the learning curve of LS. According to the data of our center, pancreatic injury after LS is mostly manifested as the increase of pancreatic enzyme in drainage fluid. According to the classification of international study group of pancreatic surgery (ISGPS), most of the pancreatic fistulas are classified as grade A, and no special treatment is needed apart from maintaining drainage tube unobstructed. Postoperative trypsin inhibitors can be used in patients with intraoperative pancreatic lesion.
3. Seroperitoneum: Attention should be paid to ensure the patency of the abdominal drainage tube, because the poor drainage of seroperitoneum may lead to abdominal infection and even the formation of abdominal abscess. If necessary, percutaneous puncture and catheterization should be performed for drainage. If postoperative monitoring of drainage fluid amylase shows that there is no fistula, no special symptoms (fever, abdominal distension, abdominal pain, etc.), and no splenic fossa effusion confirmed by imaging, the abdominal drainage tube can be removed. In our center, an orthopedic drainage tube is generally placed in the splenic fossa after

LS. In order to promote the rapid recovery of patients, if the drainage fluid is less than 10 mL or none on POD 0, with the confirmation of no pancreatic fistula, the abdominal drainage tube could be removed on POD 3.

4. Urinary tract infection: Catheter is routinely placed during LS. For high-risk patients in terms of urinary retention, they can be administrated with tamsulosin hydrochloride sustained-release capsule, combined with finasteride if necessary. The extraction of catheter for such patients is usually on POD 3 and, for others, on POD 1. Under this treatment, patients can generally urinate smoothly to avoid the secondary placement of the catheter and higher risk of urinary tract infection. Literatures [16] show that the risk of urinary tract infection will increase by about 6% in a progressive manner, for each prolonged day of catheter indwelling.
5. Pulmonary complications: In addition to common pulmonary atelectasis and its infection, there may also be left pleural effusion, which may be related to the effect of diaphragm stimulation after surgery on the postoperative diaphragmatic muscle movement. Postoperative splenic fossa effusion may also affect respiration and increase the incidence of pulmonary infection. Therefore, it is necessary to actively deal with the splenic fossa effusion. Occasionally, a large amount of pleural hydrothorax occurs, which requires ultrasound-guided positioning for thoracic puncture drainage.
6. Abdominal infection: Subphrenic infection or even subphrenic abscess is much common, which is usually associated with postoperative bleeding and distal pancreatic injury. For the fever occurring after POD 3, especially the high fever (exceeding 39 °C/102.2 °F), special precautions should be taken against the possibility of abdominal abscess. For patients with unexplained postoperative fever, abdominal color ultrasonography should be performed as soon as possible to exclude the possibility of splenic fossa effusion, hematocele, and even secondary infection.
7. Splenic fever: It refers to a fever that lasts for 2–3 weeks after splenectomy and excludes various infectious complications. Its pathogenesis is unknown, which may be related to immune factors, splenic vein embolization, and abdominal effusion. The duration is proportional to the surgical trauma. It is self-limited, generally not higher than 39 °C/102.2°2, and often regresses spontaneously within a month without treatment. If there is obvious systemic symptom, NSAIDs can be orally administered for symptomatic treatment.
8. Overwhelming postsplenectomy infection (OPSI): It was firstly reported overseas in 1952, and this infection was mostly common in children, especially in infants and young children. The infection rate is highest in patients with primary hematopathy after splenectomy. Huisheng Xia put forward OPSI diagnostic criteria in his summative speech at the second Chongqing Splenic Conference [17]: (a) a history of total splenectomy; (b) typical clinical symptoms of sudden systemic infection; (c) dermal hemorrhage spots and DIC; (d) obvious acidosis without specific localized surgical infection or abscess; (e) blood bacterial culture or smear showing positive or negative result; and (f) dual adrenal hemorrhage, visceral bleeding, etc.
9. Gastroenterol perforation: It is mainly caused by intraoperative gastric and colon injuries because of the aimless operation due to the surgeon's unclear understanding of the anatomy or poor intraoperative exposure. Sometimes, severe abdominal adhesion of the patient may also increase the risk of such injury. Once perforation occurs, the signs of peritonitis may be seen on the patient, and gastrointestinal contents may appear in the drainage tube. Oral intake of methylene blue may assist in the diagnosis. For minor perforation, the symptoms and signs of the patient are relatively mild, and adequate drainage combined with anti-infection and parenteral nutrition support can be selected; otherwise, emergent surgical exploration, drainage, suture, and fistula should be carried out.

10. Splenic vein and portal vein thrombosis: Splenic vein or portal vein thrombosis is a potentially life-threatening complication that may occur within a few months after surgery [18, 19]. It can cause ischemic necrosis of the intestine and portal hypertension. Some literatures [19, 20] reported that the incidence of portal vein thrombosis after LS is as high as 22.5–55.0%. Currently, scientists hold the idea that the risk factors are hyperfunctional coagulation, hemolytic anemia, hypersplenism, hematological malignant tumor, and splenomegaly [21]. Its clinical symptom is often non-specific, including diffusing abdominal pain, nausea, fever, intestinal obstruction, diarrhea, and decreased appetite [18, 22–24]. Generally, color ultrasound, enhanced CT scan, and magnetic resonance tomography can facilitate such diagnosis [22, 23, 25]. After the diagnosis is confirmed, LMWH or warfarin treatment should be administrated immediately, and the therapeutic dose of LMWH is maintained until discharge to obtain the good results [22]. Systemic thrombolytic therapy with streptokinase or alteplase is an alternative [26], but is rarely used. Currently, the target of warfarin treatment is to maintain the international normalized ratio (INR) between 2 and 3, with a treatment course of more than 6 months.
11. Acute pancreatitis: It is rare, mostly associated with intraoperative injury to the distal pancreas. For patients with severe postoperative abdominal pain, the possibility of this disease should be considered, and serum amylase and lipase should be detected by blood sampling in time, so as to make a definite diagnosis.
12. Jaundice, liver coma: It is rare, mostly in patients with cirrhosis complicated with portal hypertension. The prognosis of the complication is generally poor. So, we should be on high alert, focus on its prevention, and strictly control the indication of LS preoperatively.

5.7.2.2 Common Complications Associated with Laparoscopy Technology

Complications Related to Puncture

1. Vascular injury: It mainly refers to the injury caused by puncturing or tearing of abdominal vessels or larger vessels in the abdominal cavity due to technical reasons such as improper use of instruments or unclear tissue identification during veress needle or puncture sheath puncture of abdominal wall. Its occurrence rate has not been precisely reported yet, usually 0.1% or so based on the domestic and international reports. Although its overall incidence is relatively low, this kind of injury is usually an important reason leading to direct conversion to open surgery or postoperative reoperation for hemostasis. At present, our center mainly adopts the closure method, but for novices, the operation should be conducted under the guidance of an experienced laparoscopic surgeon, especially for elderly patients and patients with the thinner, looser, fatter, or thicker and tougher abdominal wall. In addition, after the operation, it is necessary to probe each puncture hole again under laparoscope carefully to see whether there is bleeding or oozing.
2. Visceral injury: It may be divided into two main types. The first type is the injury of hollow organs, including colon, small intestine, stomach, bladder, and so on. The second type is the injury of parenchymatous organs, mainly including the liver, spleen, and kidney. Due to the blind puncture with closure method, which is mainly conducted around the umbilical cord, the incidence of hollow organ injury in laparoscopic splenectomy is relatively high. However, due to the relatively low risk of puncture in other operating holes under endoscopic view, umbilical puncture must be performed with caution and excessive force shall be avoided. For patients with previous surgical history or severe abdominal adhesions, puncture should be performed by experienced laparoscopic surgeons.

Subcutaneous Emphysema

It is common in clinical practice, and most of them will not incur adverse consequences. It mainly occurs when the anatomy of abdominal wall is unclear while puncturing by veress needle or trocar. For elderly patients and patients with abdominal wall tissue relaxation, long operation time, or excessively high pneumoperitoneal pressure, the occurrence of such complication is much higher. The main preventive measures are to master the correct technique of establishing pneumoperitoneum, avoid the injection of CO_2 by veress needle in the extraperitoneal space, vertically enter the trocar into the abdominal cavity, and make sure the puncture hole should not be too large and the pneumoperitoneal pressure should be not be set too high, preferably about 13 mmHg.

Hypercapnia or Acidosis

Usually we use CO_2 to establish pneumoperitoneum. Under this constant pressure, CO_2 can be diffused into the blood through the viscera and peritoneum. When a large amount of exogenous CO_2 is absorbed into the blood, the body cannot metabolize them and hypercapnia can be formed, generally without hypoxemia. Since the duration of LS in our center is relatively short, and the pneumoperitoneal pressure is generally 13 mmHg, it will not be harmful to the body for a majority of the patients due to the buffering system of the blood and sufficient metabolism of respiratory and kidney.

Other rare complications associated with the laparoscopy technology include puncture hole infection, puncture hole hernia, pneumothorax pneumomediastinum, CO_2 gas embolism, cardiac dysfunction, deep venous congestion, or thrombosis in low extremities.

5.8 Hot Topics and Future Prospects

5.8.1 Safety and Effectiveness

LS was first reported in 1991 [1] and has been widely recognized for its low incidence of postoperative complications and good cosmetic effect. Initially, LS is mainly used in patients with hematological system disease and with normal spleen or mild splenomegaly, so LS in the treatment of hematological system diseases is as safe and feasible as open splenectomy, with even more advantages. Moreover, our data has also confirmed that compared with traditional OS, LS is a safe and effective surgical method, with all of the advantages of minimally invasive surgery. Compared with OS, LS is also reliable in the efficacy, and it has many advantages such as fewer traumas, artistic incision, less blood loss, light postoperative pain, rapid recovery of gastrointestinal function, early oral intake, fewer complications, and short hospital stay. It is undeniable that LS also has its own limitations. Currently, the possible disadvantage of LS is a relatively long time taken to extract specimens. But now there are special specimen bags, which can significantly shorten the operation time. In addition, the operation time of LS will be shortened gradually as the experience of the surgeon is accumulated. In conclusion, LS has a significant, safe, and reliable efficacy in the treatment of hematological system diseases and spleen-related diseases and has the same long-term efficacy as OS. Our data has also confirmed the safety and efficacy of laparoscopy in splenectomy, including the application on systemic lupus erythematosus (SLE) and ITP [27, 28]. With the advancement of technology and the development of laparoscopic instruments, its indications have been further broadened. Makrin et al. [29] and Tessier et al. [30] indicated that laparoscopic splenectomy is safe and feasible in the treatment of splenic benign and malignant tumors. Our data has confirmed these conclusions [3, 4] and concluded that laparoscopy is also safe and feasible in patients with splenomegaly [2, 31, 32].

5.8.2 Specimen Removal Specifications

Laparoscopic incision is small, so you need to extend the incision if you want to completely remove the spleen, which will lose the significance of minimally invasive operation. So usually we put the spleen into the specimen bag and slightly prolong the incision to 2–3 cm to extract it. Nevertheless, we should be aware that the spleen should be extracted intactly without any splenic tissues left in the abdomen or on the incision, especially for patients with splenic malignant tumor, in order to avoid metastasis in abdomen or on incision. In our center, the routine operation is using a sample bag when the spleen is taken out, which can effectively avoid incision metastasis and prevent leakage into the abdominal cavity when the spleen is crushed thus affecting the therapeutic effect of hematological system diseases or the formation of abdominal metastasis due to malignant tumors. Hence, pay attention when removing the spleen tissue to prevent sharp instruments from crushing it, so as to prevent the rupture of the sample bag leading to the leakage of fragments of the spleen tissue into the abdominal cavity. Normally, spleen tissue can be removed with fingers or atraumatic forceps [33]. It is generally believed that all specimens of the spleen can be cut up and taken out, except the splenic tumor, which should be taken out intactly. It should also be noted that different sample bags can be selected according to the size of the spleen. In addition, for patients with splenomegaly, unless the possibility of malignancy is considered, it is safe to cut the spleen in the abdominal cavity and take it out separately.

5.8.3 Future Prospects

As laparoscopic splenectomy is more and more widely used, it has become the standard operation for most of the splenic diseases, but its implementation should be based on the technology of the surgeon, experience, local hospital facilities, and the patient's specific condition. In addition, with the wide conduct of laparoscopy via Da Vinci robots, especially when it was approved by US Food and Drug Administration (FDA) in 2000, its safety has been verified and recognized [34]. Some major medical centers in China have started clinical exploration, but the Da Vinci robot-assisted system has not been widely spread yet due to its high technical requirements and high cost. It is believed that with the development of robot and laparoscopic equipment, and the continuous development of surgical technology and the reduction in related costs, there will be a broader application prospect of laparoscopic or robot-assisted splenectomy.

References

1. Delaitre B, Maignien B. Splenectomy by the laparoscopic approach: report of a case. Presse Med. 2263;20(44):1991.
2. Zhou J, Wu Z, Cai Y, et al. The feasibility and safety of laparoscopic splenectomy for massive splenomegaly: a comparative study. J Surg Res. 2011;171(1):55–60.
3. Meng LW, Li YB, Peng B, et al. The application of laparoscopic technology for splenic benign tumor. Chin J HBS. 2017;23(4):251–4.
4. Meng LW, Cai H, Cai YQ, et al. The treatment experience of laparoscopic technology for splenic malignant tumor. Chin J BM Clin Med Gen Surg. 2016;23(04):429–33.
5. Knauer EM, Ailawadi G, Yahanda A, et al. 101 laparoscopic splenectomies for the treatment of benign and malignant hematologic disorders. Am J Surg. 2003;186(5):500–4.
6. Habermalz B, Sauerland S, Decker G, et al. Laparoscopic splenectomy: the clinical practice guidelines of the European Association for Endoscopic Surgery (EAES). Surg Endosc. 2008;22(4):821–48.
7. Yang F. Interpretation of guidelines for the clinical application of antimicrobial drugs (2015). Chin J Clin ID. 2016;9(5):390–3.
8. Wu Z, Zhou J, Li J, et al. The feasibility of laparoscopic splenectomy for ITP patients without preoperative platelet transfusion. Hepato-Gastroenterology. 2012;59(113):81–5.
9. Chen X, Peng B, Cai Y, et al. Laparoscopic splenectomy for patients with immune thrombocytopenia and very low platelet count: is platelet transfusion necessary? J Surg Res. 2011;170(2):225–32.
10. Cai Y, Liu X, Peng B. Should we routinely transfuse platelet for immune thrombocytopenia patients with platelet count less than 10×10^9/L who underwent laparoscopic splenectomy? World J Surg. 2014;38(9):2267–72.
11. Harold KL, Pollinger H, Matthews BD, et al. Comparison of ultrasonic energy, bipolar thermal energy, and vascular clips for the hemostasis of small-, medium-, and large-sized arteries. Surg Endosc. 2003;17(8):1228–30.
12. Li CL, Chen SR, Li JB, et al. Detection of drainage fluid after laparoscopic splenectomy and its value. Chin J Surg MI. 2009;9(4):339–41.

13. Jiang HC, Qiao HQ. Splenic surgery. Shenyang: Liaoning Science and Technology Publishing House; 2007.
14. Bassi C, Marchegiani G, Dervenis C, et al. The 2016 update of the International Study Group (ISGPS) definition and grading of postoperative pancreatic fistula: 11 Years After. Surgery. 2017;161(3):584–91.
15. Chand B, Walsh RM, Ponsky J, et al. Pancreatic complications following laparoscopic splenectomy. Surg Endosc. 2001;15(11):1273–6.
16. Nazarko L. Reducing the risk of catheter-related urinary tract infection. Br J Nurs. 2008;17(16): 1002–6.
17. Xia SS. Study of spleen function and progress of splenic surgery. Gen Surg Clin. 1989;6(5):265–71.
18. Svensson M, Wiren M, Kimby E, et al. Portal vein thrombosis is a common complication following splenectomy in patients with malignant haematological diseases. Eur J Haematol. 2006;77(3):203–9.
19. Pietrabissa A, Moretto C, Antonelli G, et al. Thrombosis in the portal venous system after elective laparoscopic splenectomy. Surg Endosc. 2005;19(10):1420–1.
20. Ikeda M, Sekimoto M, Takiguchi S, et al. High incidence of thrombosis of the portal venous system after laparoscopic splenectomy: a prospective study with contrast-enhanced CT scan. Ann Surg. 2005;241(2):208–16.
21. Ikeda M, Sekimoto M, Takiguchi S, et al. Total splenic vein thrombosis after laparoscopic splenectomy: a possible candidate for treatment. Am J Surg. 2007;193(1):21–5.
22. Romano F, Caprotti R, Conti M, et al. Thrombosis of the splenoportal axis after splenectomy. Langenbeck's Arch Surg. 2006;391(5):483–8.
23. Winslow ER, Brunt LM, Drebin JA, et al. Portal vein thrombosis after splenectomy. J Am Coll Surg. 2002;184(6):631–5.
24. van't Riet M, Burger JW, van Muiswinkel JM, et al. Diagnosis and treatment of portal vein thrombosis following splenectomy. Br J Surg. 2000;87(9):1229–33.
25. Loring LA, Panicek DM, Karpeh MS. Portal system thrombosis after splenectomy for neoplasm or chronic hematologic disorder: is routine surveillance imaging necessary? J Comput Assist Tomogr. 1998;22(22):856–60.
26. Watson DI, Coventry BJ, Chin T, et al. Laparoscopic versus open splenectomy for immune thrombocytopenic purpura. Surgery. 1997;121(1):18–22.
27. Zhou J, Wu Z, Zhou Z, et al. Efficacy and safety of laparoscopic splenectomy in thrombocytopenia secondary to systemic lupus erythematosus. Clin Rheumatol. 2013;32(8):1131–8.
28. Peng B, Du JP, Niu T, et al. The application of laparoscopic splenectomy for idiopathic thrombocytopenic purpura. World Chin Med. 2006;21(3):440–1.
29. Makrin V, Avital S, White I, et al. Laparoscopic splenectomy for solitary splenic tumors. Surg Endosc. 2008;22(9):2009–12.
30. Tessier DJ, Pierce RA, Brunt LM, et al. Laparoscopic splenectomy for splenic masses. Surg Endosc. 2008;22(9):2062–6.
31. Cai YQ, Zhou J, Chen XD, et al. Laparoscopic splenectomy is an effective and safe intervention for hypersplenism secondary to liver cirrhosis. Surg Endosc. 2011;25(12):3791–7.
32. Cai Y, Liu X, Peng B. A novel method for laparoscopic splenectomy in the setting of hypersplenism secondary to liver cirrhosis: ten years' experience. World J Surg. 2014;38(11):2934–9.
33. Katkhouda N, Waldrep DJ, Feinstein D, et al. Unresolved issues in laparoscopic splenectomy. Am J Surg. 1996;172(5):585–9.
34. Stafford AT, Walsh RM. Robotic surgery of the pancreas: the current state of the art. J Surg Oncol. 2015;112(3):289–94.

6 Single Incision Laparoscopic Splenectomy (SILS)

Shuodong Wu, Runwen Liu, and Ying Fan

6.1 Background

Laparoscopic splenectomy is widely applied in clinical practice currently [1]. However, the operative technique and key points of single incision laparoscopic splenectomy (SILS) are different from those of laparoscopic splenectomy. Meanwhile, the spleen has abundant vascularity and brittle texture and is vulnerable to hemorrhage, which leads to difficulties in operation [2]. In 2009, Barbaros [3] firstly reported successful SILS in two patients with immune thrombocytopenic purpura (ITP). Since then, some scholars have reported cases of successful use of SILS for splenic diseases successively [4, 5]. In 2011, Second Department of General Surgery, Shengjing Hospital, Affiliated to China Medical University completed the first case of SILS for traumatic splenic rupture in the world [6]; in 2020, it performed transumbilical SILS combined with esophagogastric fundus pericardial vasectomy for cirrhotic portal hypertension and reported this operation on international journal firstly [7]. In 2013, Fan Ying et al. conducted a systematic meta-analysis and drew a conclusion that SILS has much more viability and safety compared with multi-incision laparoscopic splenectomy, with a better cosmetic result [8]. With the development of laparoscope and its technology, there is an increase in articles reporting SILS.

6.2 Indications and Contraindications

SILS was first used for the treatment of diseases of the blood system, especially for the treatment of ITP [9]. With the improvement of surgical skills and the usage of high-definition laparoscope, ultrasonic scalpel, and Endo-GIA stapler, the indications of SILS have been widened gradually. Currently, the indications of SILS are considered as follows.

6.2.1 Indications of SILS

1. Traumatic splenic rupture
2. Splenic benign tumors such as hemangiomas and hamartomas
3. Splenic cyst
4. Hematological system diseases, e.g., hereditary spherocytosis, refractory immune thrombocytopenic purpura, and autoimmune hemolytic anemia (AIHA)
5. Cirrhotic portal hypertension, with normal-sized spleen

S. Wu (✉) · Y. Fan
Shengjing Hospital of China Medical University, Shenyang, China

R. Liu
West China Hospital, Sichuan University, Chengdu, China

B. Peng (ed.), *Laparoscopic Surgery of the Spleen*, https://doi.org/10.1007/978-981-16-1216-9_6

6.2.2 Relative Contradictions of SILS

1. Pathological spleen led by portal hypertension. The Medical Center of Loyola University Chicago has listed portal hypertension with pathological spleen as a contradiction of SILS [10]. Some scholars believe that it is safe and effective to perform LS for portal hypertension with pathological spleen [11].
2. Splenomegaly. Some scholars consider that it is a contradiction for LS if the spleen with an interpole length of 25 cm or one that crosses the midline or enters the pelvis [12].
3. Severe perisplenitis, vascular or anatomical disorder

6.2.3 Absolute Contradictions of SILS

1. Aged patients, with other underlying diseases, intolerant to surgery
2. Severe impairment of blood coagulation, which is difficult to correct in medicine
3. Splenic malignant tumors, pregnancy splenic abscess, etc.

In a word, the indications of SILS should be handled according to the experience and skill of the surgeon, and it is critical to guarantee a safe surgery with less or no complications [13].

6.3 Preoperative Assessment and Preparation

Preoperative assessment and preparation mainly include skin preparation, biochemical examination, gastrointestinal preparation, and medicine preparation.

6.3.1 Skin Preparation in the Field of Operation

Before the operation, shave the hair above the pubis and clean the umbilical region, in order to reduce the probability of local infection in the incision.

6.3.2 Routine Biochemical Tests

Examine the blood routine, coagulating time and prothrombin time, to understand the coagulation status of the patient. If the patient's platelet (PLT) is less than 20×10^9/L, preoperative infusion of whole blood or 4–16 U platelet suspension should be carried out to prevent intraoperative hemorrhage or wound bleeding.

6.3.3 Gastrointestinal Preparation

Patients should have fasted for 12 h and have been deprived from water for 4 h preoperatively to prevent the occurrence of asphyxiation, aspiration pneumonia, and postoperative ventosity due to intraoperative nausea and vomiting. Insert gastric tube and carry out continuous gastrointestinal decompression preoperatively and evacuate gastric contents to remit flatulence.

6.3.4 Medicine Preparation

Patients with immune thrombocytopenic purpura should be administrated with hydrocortisone 3 days before surgery at a dose of 100–300 mg/day, to prevent the occurrence of hemolysis crisis; patients with liver cirrhosis should be provided with proper treatment to protect liver and correct hypoproteinemia and liver function. If patients are suffering from ascites, the operation can be performed after ascites retrogression.

6.4 Surgical Procedures

6.4.1 Surgical Position and Surgeon Position (Fig. 6.1)

Surgical position: After the success of general anesthesia, outstretch the patient's upper limbs both sides horizontally and lower limbs

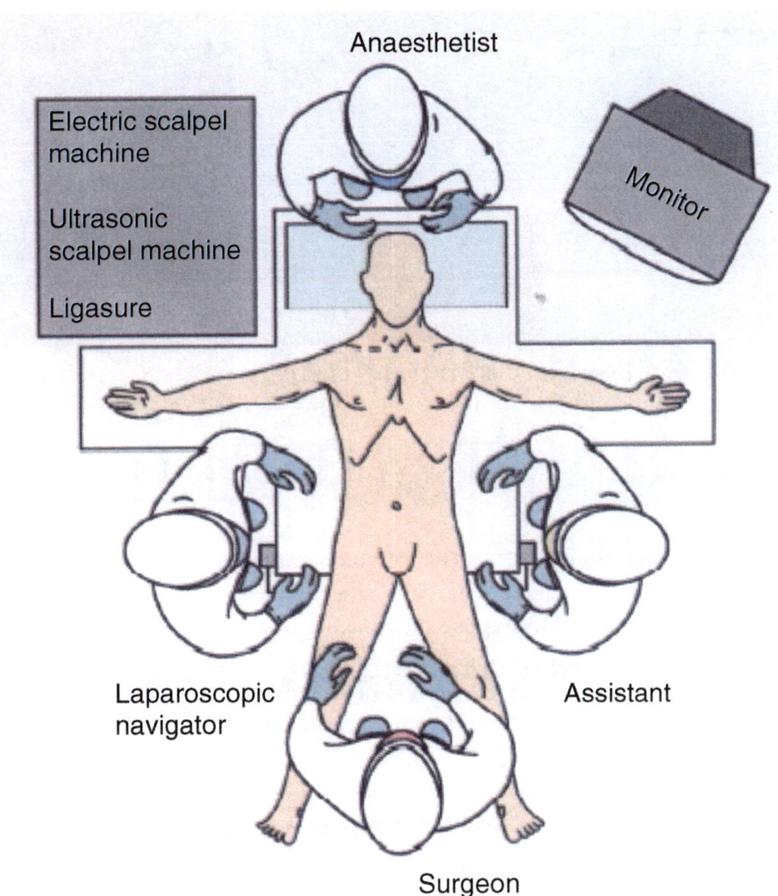

Fig. 6.1 Surgical position and surgeon position

for 30–45°, and pad the left shoulder-back for about 15–20°.

Surgeon position and device placement: The surgeon stands between the legs of the patient, the laparoscopic navigator usually stands on the right side of the patient, and the assistant stands on the left side; the monitor is placed to the outside of the patient's left shoulder. Compared with porous incision, SILS is more difficult to perform, with fewer devices used, so it is necessary to use body position and gravity to expose the field.

6.4.2 Main Steps

1. Place the trocar and establish the pneumoperitoneum. Make an incision about 2 cm long through the umbilical region, keeping the fascia layer intact and avoid air leakage during the pneumoperitoneum. After successful pneumoperitoneum, perform puncture with 10 mm trocar at the bottom of the incision, insert the laparoscope to confirm the feasibility of single-incision laparoscopic surgery. Then place 5 mm trocar and 12 mm trocar on the upper edge of the surgical incision, arranging the three trocars in an inverse triangle (Fig. 6.2). Then, insert grasping forceps, ultrasonic scalpel, or LigaSure into 5 mm trocar and 12 mm trocar, respectively, for tissue separation and coagulation [14]. Set CO_2 pneumoperitoneum pressure at 12–14 mmHg.
2. Dissect the spleen. First, dissociate the gastrocolic ligament to expose the pancreas. Continue to dissociate the splenogastric ligament, and cut off the short gastric vessels with ultrasonic scalpel. Then dissociate the splenocolic ligament by ultrasound scalpel, avoiding

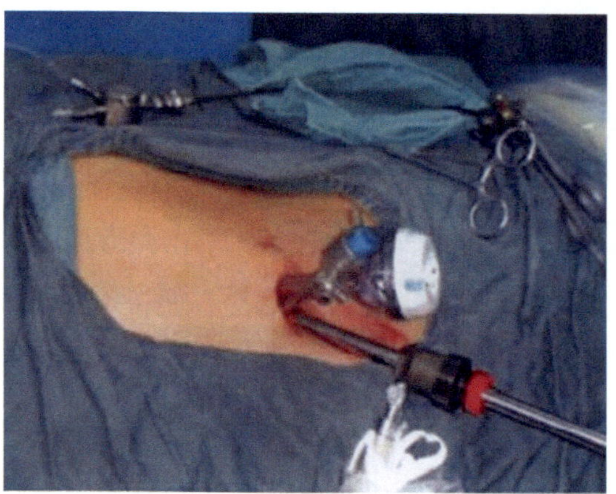

Fig. 6.2 Trocar of SILS arranged into an inverse triangle

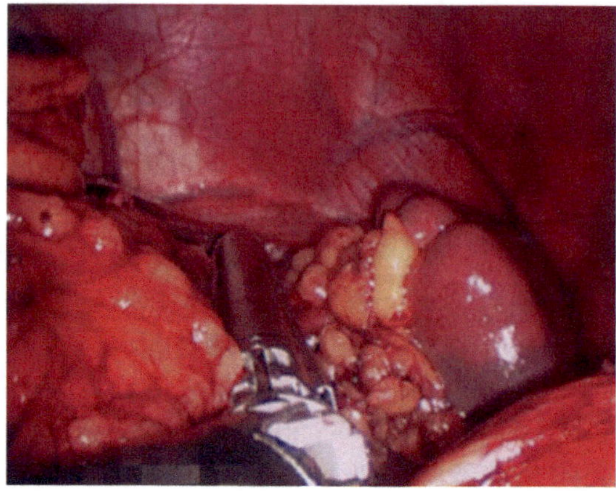

Fig. 6.3 Cut off the ligated splenic pedicle by Endo-GIA under laparoscope

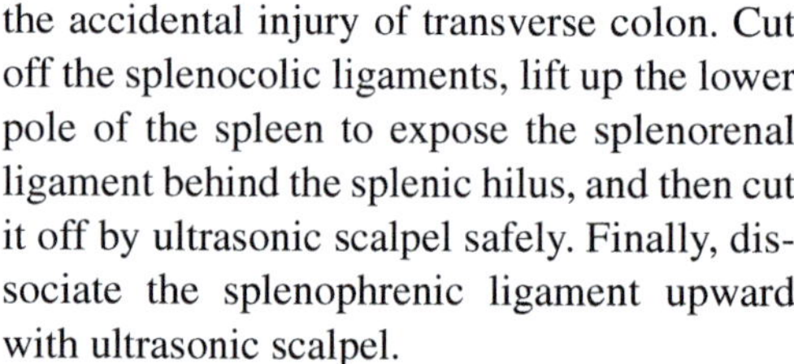

the accidental injury of transverse colon. Cut off the splenocolic ligaments, lift up the lower pole of the spleen to expose the splenorenal ligament behind the splenic hilus, and then cut it off by ultrasonic scalpel safely. Finally, dissociate the splenophrenic ligament upward with ultrasonic scalpel.

3. Dispose of splenic pedicle. Use ultrasound scalpel with LigaSure to carefully dissociate the peritoneum of the splenic hilum, and then expose the pancreatic tail and protect it. Dissect the splenic pedicle at the splenic hilum after dissociating in the front of the pancreatic tail. Place a 60 mm linear Endo-GIA through a 12 mm trocar to close the splenic pedicle (Fig. 6.3), to complete hemostasia and splenectomy. In patients with splenomegaly or with difficulty in exposing or dissecting splenic pedicle, hand-assisted laparoscopic splenectomy can be used in laparoscopic splenectomy, to dispose of the splenic arteries and veins and remove the spleen under direct vision.
4. Take specimen. Place the spleen into the sample bag placed via 12 mm trocar. Due to the limitation of single-incision laparoscope, load the spleen into the sample bag with the change of body position (Fig. 6.4). This process requires skilled laparoscopic technique and sufficient patience. Tighten the mouth of the specimen bag, clamp it, and drag it into the trocar. Pull it out together with the trocar. Expand the mouth of the specimen bag, and extract splenic tissues in batches by sponge forceps.

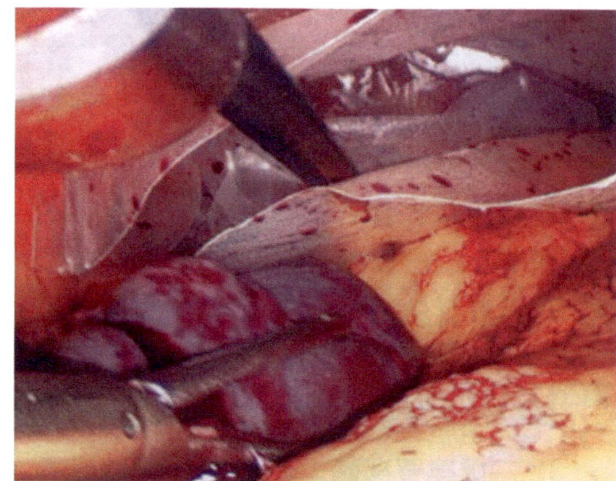

Fig. 6.4 Load splenic tissue into the sample bag

5. Place the drainage tube. Rinse locally and suck the abdominal hemoperitoneum. Detect whether there is bleeding or leakage, and after the check of the gauze and other instruments, retain a drainage tube in the spleen fossa, which should be extracted through the umbilical cord (Figs. 6.5 and 6.6).

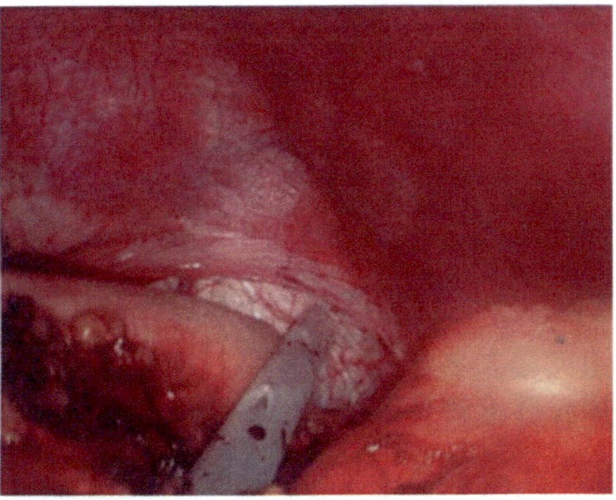

Fig. 6.5 Placement of the drainage tube: retaining a drainage tube in spleen fossa

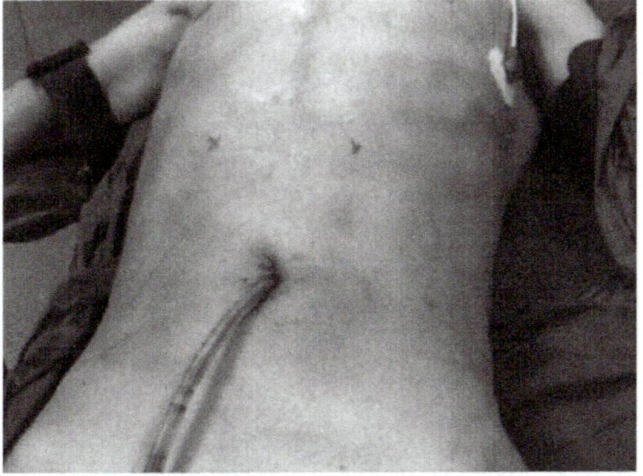

Fig. 6.6 Placement of the drainage tube: drainage via the umbilical cord

6.5 Key Surgical Techniques

6.5.1 Techniques for Dissociation of the Spleen via Single-Incision

The dissociation of the perisplenic ligaments is an important step in the process of SILS. We should pay attention to the following points [15]:

1. The dissociation of the upper pole of the spleen and the splenophrenic ligament is a difficult part, given the fact that the spleen is adjacent to the gastric wall and the diaphragm, with short gastric vessels running inside, which is difficult to be exposed, and the operating space is narrow. If handled improperly, bleeding and gastric wall and diaphragmatic injury can be caused. If the gastric distension occurs, take out gastric contents via gastric tube; lift the upper pole of the spleen gently with aspirer by left hand, making that there is moderate tension between spleen, the stomach fundus, and the diaphragm; then dissect the serous layer of the splenogastric ligament by ultrasonic scalpel to release the ligament and expand the gap; dissociate short gastric vessels; and after the clear exposal, clip and cut off the short gastric vessels by vessel clips and ultrasonic scalpel, respectively, so as to avoid the injury of the stomach and the spleen. For the patients with portal hypertension, cut off varicose veins by vessel clips in avoidance of intraoperative and postoperative bleeding.
2. Some patients with portal hypertension have severe retroperitoneal varicose veins. When operating on such patients, perform as close as possible to the spleen during the process of dissociating the splenorenal ligament, for avoiding incorrect surgical layer. After entering the anterior renal space, avoid massive bleeding caused by the injury of retroperitoneal varicose veins.

6.5.2 Treatment of Splenic Artery

After dissociating the perisplenic ligaments, look for and identify the splenic artery at the upper margin of the distal pancreas and ligate it after its dissociation, which is a critical step especially in patients with portal hypertension. After the ligation of splenic artery, due to the lack of the splenic perfusion, the texture of the spleen becomes soft, with its slightly reduced size and the reduction of the hemorrhage it would be, making the operation easier and facilitating the later steps. If it is difficult to find the splenic artery at the upper margin of the distal pancreas, follow the common hepatic artery and dissociate to the left to identify the splenic artery.

6.5.3 Treatment of Splenic Hilum

Treatment of splenic hilum is one of the difficulties during the SILS, and there are a variety of surgical plans in the medical centers at home and abroad, which can be summarized into two categories:

1. Ligament of secondary branches of splenic pedicle. Use silk thread or vascular clip to clip the trunk and branches of the splenic artery and vein in order, and then ligate the splenic pedicle completely.
2. Ligament of primary branches of splenic pedicle. Create tunnels on the front and rear of the pancreatic tail near the splenic hilus, and then use Endo-GIA to ligate splenic vessels completely.

The first method is to dissect and cut off splenic vessels, respectively, with a precise and reliable hemostasis, but it is more time-consuming; for the patient with obesity, tortuosity, and expansion of splenic vessels, and with peri-pancreatic tail adhesions, this method for dissecting vessels is more difficult to be carried out, and it is more vulnerable to hemorrhage in the process of dissection. Thus, it is advisable to apply the second method on such patient, for its sufficiency on dissecting and its avoidance on injuring pancreatic tail and stomach. In addition, the thickness of the staple cartridge is selected according to the thickness of the tissue. For example, if the splenoportal tissue is more abundant and wider, with tortuous splenic vessels, the whole tissue can be ligated with silk thread first and then cut with Endo-GIA after the spleen pedicle is narrowed in order to ensure the ligamental effect. It should be emphasized that it is vital to confirm whether the staple cartridge is not clipped on vascular clip, suspension band, gauze strips, and so on before starting the Endo-GIA, so as to avoid poor closure leading to massive hemorrhage [16–18].

6.5.4 Techniques for Specimen Removal

After the total splenectomy, put the specimens into a disposable sample bag, remove it from the splenic fossa, wash the wound surface with warm saline, and check the presence of bleeding and pancreatic lesions again. Meanwhile, the presence of surrounding accessory spleen should be checked. Apart from the complete removal of the malignant splenic specimens, other types of spleen specimens can be chopped before removed. It should be noted that different sizes of sample bags can be selected according to the size of the specimen, and the bag should be anti-tension to avoid the splenic implantation after the rupture of the specimen belt, which will affect the surgical effect.

6.6 Special Intraoperative Circumstances and Handling Skills

6.6.1 Intraoperative Hemorrhage

The spleen is deeply located with brittle texture and abundant blood supply, which can easily lead to bleeding during laparoscopic splenectomy. If there is an accidental hemorrhage during the operation, stay calm at first, use a small gauze strip to compress the bleeding site, and then identify and handle the bleeding site carefully after cleared by an aspirator. If the hemorrhage is difficult to be dealt with under laparoscope, it shall be transferred to hand assistance or open surgery. Timely transferring to open surgery does not mean the failure of laparoscopic surgery, but the better maintenance of the patient's life based on the principle of "life first." In order to prevent bleeding during laparoscopic splenectomy, the following methods can be summarized after consulting a large number of domestic and foreign literatures [19–22]:

1. Strictly control the indications of surgery, and check the preoperative coagulation function routinely.
2. During the operation, the patient should be carefully operated with clear anatomical layers and operative fields to prevent iatrogenic hemorrhage. During the operation, the force to pull perisplenal ligament should be moderate with the correct method. The spleen cannot be directly clamped; instead, place gauze blocks on the head of the aspirator and use the aspirator to expose the spleen by poking, carrying apart, pushing, elevating, and any other gentle way. Usually, during the operation, dispose of the perisplenic ligament first, then the short gastric vessels, and last the splenic pedicle. A few relevant articles suggest that it is not necessary to cut off the short gastric vessels completely at one time if there is difficulty in disposing of the short gastric vessels; after handling the spleen pedicle, cut off the remaining short gastric vessels [20].
3. Ultrasound scalpel is mainly used for dissociation and dissection during the operation. The ultrasonic scalpel has many advantages such as convenience to use, high operation accuracy, good coagulation function, clear separation of surrounding tissues, low probability of accidental injury to surrounding tissues, and so on.
4. Timely transfer to open surgery during the operation does not mean the failure of the operation; instead, it is good for the better maintenance of the patient's life based on the principle of "life first."
5. The drainage tube placed in the splenic fossa after surgery can timely detect the splenic pedicle bleeding, which makes decisive measures to carry out to dispose of bleeding and to save patient's life in time.
6. The operative field should be fully exposed intraoperatively, and the surgical operation should be carried out step by step. Attention should be paid to the possible presence of the accessory spleen, which must be removed simultaneously if detected.

6.6.2 Adjacent Organ Injury

Given the unclear tissue exposure during the operation, the nearby stomach and colon might be injured or perforated. According to the intraoperative conditions, primary suture or building fistula is selected.

6.7 Postoperative Management and Prevention and Treatment of Complications

6.7.1 Routine Postoperative Care

1. The patient should be kept in a supine position after the operation. In order to prevent the patient's vomit from blocking the trachea, the patient's head can be turned to one side.
2. Closely observe the patient's vital signs, measure blood pressure, respiration, and pulse every hour, and constantly monitor the patient's temperature and oxygen saturation. Observe the patient's change of mental state and psychological and physical appearance.
3. Observe the patient's abdominal signs, paying attention to whether the patient has abdominal pain or distension.
4. After the postoperative recovery of intestinal function, remove the gastric tube; instruct the patient to gradually intake liquid and/or semi-liquid food. Due to the less traumatic of laparoscopic splenectomy, it has marginal impact on the human gastrointestinal system; thus the recovery of gastrointestinal function is rapid, the gastric tube can usually be removed a day or so postoperatively. Many patients will develop nausea in the short term after the operation, which is due to the use of pneumoperitoneum and anesthesia intraoperatively; intramuscular injection of metoclopramide can be applied.
5. Closely observe the incision and abdominal drainage tube. Observe whether there is seepage or bleeding at the incision; replace the

dressing on time to keep the incision hygienic. Observe the quantity and quality of the abdominal drainage fluid, record the drainage volume each hour on the day of operation, and take notice on the patency of the drainage tube. If there's active hemorrhage or oozing of blood in abdominal cavity, drainage fluid will increase; detect and treat it timely. The drainage tube can be removed when the drainage fluid is reduced to less than 20 mL/day.

6.7.2 Common Postoperative Complications and Their Prevention and Treatment

Previous studies have shown that the occurrence of complications of open splenectomy ranges from 5% to 60%, mainly including hemorrhage, pancreatic tail injury, and pulmonary complications, while the incidence of complications of splenectomy for patients with splenomegaly and splenic malignancy ranges from 40% to 60% [23, 24]. With the popularization of laparoscopic splenectomy, the incidence of complications is significantly lower than that of open splenectomy due to the minimally invasive, high-definition, enlarged operative field and delicate and gentle operation. However, the complications of laparoscopic splenectomy cannot be completely avoided due to the complicated anatomy and variability of the spleen, especially the pathologic spleen coincides with coagulation dysfunction and ultra-splenomegaly.

1. Gastric fistula, intestinal fistula, and pancreatic fistula. The internal injuries are not only caused by puncture cannula or pneumoperitoneum needle, but also related to surgical operation. Improper use of electric cauterization can cause iatrogenic gastric, colon, and pancreatic injuries [25]. If the dissection of splenocolic or splenogastric ligament is too close to the colon, the thermoelectric effect produced by cautery hook can cause gastric and colon injury, resulting in delayed gastrointestinal perforation. When the gastric wall is clamped, it can cause the ischemia and necrosis of the gastric wall, resulting in gastric fistula. Given the pancreatic tail is close to the spleen, if the dissociation of splenic vessels is far away from the splenic hilus, the pancreatic tail will be easily damaged, causing pancreatic fistula. Electrocoagulation hemostasis at the splenic hilum under non-direct vision may cause severe bleeding; therefore, in electrocoagulation, electrotomy, clipping, and cutting off of the splenogastric, splenocolic, and splenophrenic ligaments, the maintenance of a certain tension is needed. Such procedure should change into mobilization of lower pole of spleen should close to spleen, do not damage the colon, stomach, or diaphragm [26]. In the dissection of splenic hilum, the sharpness dissection via ultrasonic knife should be adopted as much as possible to prevent the tearing of the spleen capsule. Pay attention to checking serum amylase postoperatively, to timely detect and handle pancreatic injury [27].
2. Postoperative bleeding. Postoperative bleeding should be disposed of immediately if found; secondary operation (endoscopy or laparoscopy) is needed if non-surgical treatment to hemorrhage cannot control bleeding.
3. Thrombosis in mesenteric blood vessels, deep vein of lower limbs, or spleen-portal vein. Thrombosis is a complication with low incidence; the reason may be associated with platelet rising velocity [28, 29]; therefore, constantly monitoring the change of platelet and coagulation is needed, and if it is necessary, use medication to regulate platelet and coagulation, which helps to reduce the incidence of the complication of thrombosis. If the platelet increases to 600×10^9/L, medication can be appropriately used to reduce the counting of platelets. Assisting patients on off-bed activity is an effective way to prevent thrombosis. If thrombosis occurs in lower limbs, nurses should instruct patients to lie down and elevate the affected limb.
4. Postoperative fever and infection. Most of the patients will have fever within 3 days after operation. There are two causes of rising body temperature, one is splenic fever, which can be diagnosed if infective diagnoses are

excluded, then carry out antipyretic treatments. Generally, liver function plays a more important role in splenic fever, it is important to detect and improve liver function perioperatively. In the second case, if the body temperature exceeds 39 °C (102 °F) and lasts for more than 3 days, the occurrence of postoperative infection should be taken into accounts. Postoperative splenic fossa fluid infection is prone to occur; in this case, find the infection sources out in time, and appropriate usage of antibiotics and puncture drainage should be used for treatment. Some patients will also suffer from pulmonary, incision, and abdominal cavity infection postoperatively. For the prevention of pulmonary infection, patients should be informed to pay attention to respiratory function exercise before surgery, atomization inhalation treatment should be carried out twice a day postoperatively, and guide patients to cough effectively. Abdominal infection is usually caused by peritoneal effusion; drainage tube should be placed in the splenic fossa to extract the effusion in time. Take good care of the skin around the orifice of the drainage tube. Timely change of dressing can keep the incision dry and clean.

5. Complications related to accessory spleen. Velanovich et al. [30] reported that five cases of patients with hematology disease underwent laparoscopic accessory splenectomy due to the presence of accessory spleen after splenectomy, of which two cases were significantly improved. The occurrence rate of accessory spleen is 15–20%; among the patients with hematology disease, such probability is as high as 30% [31]. CT and ultrasound examination should be completed preoperatively; the exploration should be carried out first after the laparoscopy enters the abdomen, and the accessory spleen should be resected when it is found. It would be difficult to find the accessory spleen after splenectomy for the accessory spleen is mainly on the splenic hilum, pancreatic tail, omentum, mesentery, and perisplenic ligament. During hand-assisted laparoscopic splenectomy, the accessory spleen could be found with finger with sensitive tackle to prevent omission. When the specimen is being taken out, the legacy of the accessory spleen or autologous transplantation of splenic tissue fragments may lead to surgical failure. Due to its own limitations, SILS is more likely to cause omissions if there is slightly negligent. During the operation, put splenic specimens into the bag. Then fasten the mouth of the bag, which should be put out of the abdominal wall, and finally cut up the specimens with gyno uterine rotation cutter or break it with oval forceps, remembering that the sample bag should be avoided to be perforated.

6.8 Hot Topics and Future Prospects

6.8.1 Advantages of SILS

Traditional LS makes four incisions in the patient's umbilicus and upper abdomen, while SILS only makes a 3 cm incision in the fold of the umbilicus. After healing, due to the cover of the fold of the navel, the surgical scar is almost difficult to be detected, which has an obvious psychological comfort on patients, especially on young and unmarried patients.

6.8.2 Disadvantages of SILS

Given the parallel arrangement between the equipment and the mutual interference between surgeon and laparoscopic navigator in SILS, surgical instruments cannot be fully unfolded, which leads to an apparent "chopsticks effect" and a higher difficulty compared to LS, so its indication has certain limitation, especially in the early stages of the operation; patients with no abdominal surgery history and no obesity with normal-sized spleen and strong desire of beauty simultaneously are suitable to such operation. This technique has a unique learning curve, requiring good cooperation between the laparoscopic navigator and the surgeon, lessening interference with surgical instruments while ensuring a clear view. Therefore, the requirements for the surgical are stringent.

6.8.3 Future Prospects

SILS is safe and feasible if its indications and contradictions are handled properly [32]. At home and abroad, the research for robot-assisted splenectomy will be much more mature; the multiangular rotation of the robot arm can overcome the "chopsticks effects" in a single-incisional operation. A few large- and medium-sized hospitals have put it into clinical use gradually, which will then be carried out by primary hospitals. Presently, the top priority is given to train a large number of skilled endoscopic surgeons, followed by the continuous development of advanced laparoscopic equipment to keep up with the development of surgical needs. It is believed that with the continuous development of society, science and technology, the continuous update of laparoscopic instruments, and the continuous deepening of LS research, SILS will play a greater role in the research and clinical application of splenic surgery.

References

1. Habermalz B, Sauerland S, Decker G, et al. Laparoscopic splenectomy: the clinical practice guidelines of the European Association for Endoscopic Surgery (EAES). Surg Endosc. 2008;22(4):821–48.
2. Podolsky ER, Curcillo PG. II. Single port access (SPA) surgery: a 24-month experience. J Gastrointest Surg. 2010;14(5):759–67.
3. Barbaros U, Dinccag A. Single incision laparoscopic splenectomy: the first two cases. J Gastrointest Surg. 2009;13(8):1520–3.
4. Malladi P, Hungness E, Nagle A. Single access laparoscopic splenectomy. JSLS. 2009;13(4):601–4.
5. Targarona EM, Lima MB, Balague C, et al. Single-port splenectomy: current update and controversies. J Minim Access Surg. 2011;7(1):61–4.
6. Fan Y, Wu SD, Siwo EA. Emergency Transumbilical Single-Incision Laparoscopic Splenectomy for the Treatment of Traumatic Rupture of the Spleen: Report of the First Case and Literature Review. Surg Innov. 2011;18(2):185–8.
7. Jing K, Shuo-Dong W, Ying F. Transumbilical single-incision laparoscopy surgery splenectomy plus pericaudial devascularization in one case with portal hypertension: the first report. Surg Innov. 2013;20(6):21–4.
8. Fan Y, Wu SD, Kong J, et al. Feasibility and safety of single-incision laparoscopic splenectomy: a systematic review. J Surg Res. 2014;186(1):354–62.
9. Dionigi R, Boni L, Rausei S, et al. History of splenectomy. Int J Surg. 2013;11(1):42–3.
10. Fisichella PM, Wong YM, Pappas SG, et al. Laparoscopic splenectomy: perioperative management, surgical technique, and results. J Gastrointest Surg. 2014;18(2):404–10.
11. Cai Y, Liu X. Few comments on "laparoscopic splenectomy: perioperative management, surgical technique, and results". J Gastrointest Surg. 2014;18(10):1881.
12. Koshenkov VP, Nemeth ZH, Carter MS. Laparoscopic splenectomy: outcome and efficacy for massive and supramassive spleens. Am J Surg. 2012;203(4):517–22.
13. Bhandarkar DS, Katara AN, Mittal G, et al. Prevention and management of complications of laparoscopic splenectomy. Indian J Surg. 2011;73(5):324–30.
14. Hu SY, Zhang JL. Laparoscopic Splenectomy. Chinese J Pract Surg. 1998;18(05):263–5.
15. Zhan HX, Hu SY. The key points and difficulties of laparoscopic splenectomy. J Laparoscopic Surg. 2016;8(21):567–9.
16. Lv GY, Sun XD, Wang YC, et al. Experience of clinical application of laparoscopic splenectomy in hypersplenism of portal hypertension. Chin J Hepatobiliary Surg. 2010;16(12):928–30.
17. Wang GY, Liu YH, Lv GY, et al. Application of two-step dissection of vessel closure system in secondary splenic pedicle ligation in laparoscopic splenectomy. Chin J Surg. 2008;46(19):1457–9.
18. Wang GY, Liu YH, Lv GY, et al. The summarization of the experience of laparoscopic splenectomy with two-step dissection for secondary splenic pedicle ligation in 105 cases. Chin J Surg. 2010;48(24):1894–5.
19. Weng C, Wu SD, Fan Y, et al. Clinical application of transumbilical single incision laparoscopic splenectomy: experience of single center (with video). Chin General Surg. 2013;7(02):20–3.
20. Hu SY, Zhang GY, Qi YL, et al. Laparoscopic splenectomy: a report of 43 cases. Chin J Pract Surg. 2004;24(2):109–10.
21. Zhang GY, Wang L, Liu SZ, et al. A report of 6 cases of hybrid transumbilical single incision laparoscopic splenectomy. J Laparoscopic Surg. 2013;18(03):163–7.
22. Liu CZ, Hu SY, Zhang GY, et al. A comparative study of laparoscopic splenectomy and open splenectomy. Chin J General Surg. 2006;21(11):834.
23. Yong F, Chen W, Lan P, Youcheng Z. Applications of laparoscopic technique in spleen surgery. Eur Rev Med Pharmacol Sci. 2014;18(12):1713–6.

24. Patel NY, Chilsen AM, Mathiason MA, et al. Outcomes and complications after splenectomy for hematologic disorders. Am J Surg. 2012;204(6):1014–9.
25. Hu RJ, Qin HJ, Cheng G, et al. Some discussion on laparoscopic splenectomy. J Hepatopancreatob Surg. 2015;27(02):143–5.
26. Zhu JF. Laparoscopic splenectomy. J Pract Clin Med. 2003;7(05):411–3.
27. Chand B, Walsh RM, Ponsky J, et al. Pancreatic complications following laparoscopic splenectomy. Surg Endosc. 2001;15(11):1273–6.
28. Xiang JX, Liu XM, Liu P, et al. Risk factors for portal vein thrombosis and its transition to open surgery in laparoscopic splenectomy. Abdom Surg. 2015;28(6):389–93.
29. Franciosi C, Romano F, Caprotti R, et al. Splenoportal thrombosis as a complication after laparoscopic splenectomy. J Laparoendosc Adv Surg Tech A. 2002;12(4):273–6.
30. Velanovich V, Shurafa M. Laparoscopic excision of accessory spleen. Am J Surg. 2000;180(1):62–4.
31. Katkhouda N, Hurwitz MB, Rivera RT, et al. Laparoscopic splenectomy: outcome and efficacy in 103 Consecutive Patients. Ann Surg. 1998;228(4):568–78.
32. Hong DF. Surgical techniques for laparoscopic splenectomy. J Hepatobiliary Surg. 2010;18(6):406–8.

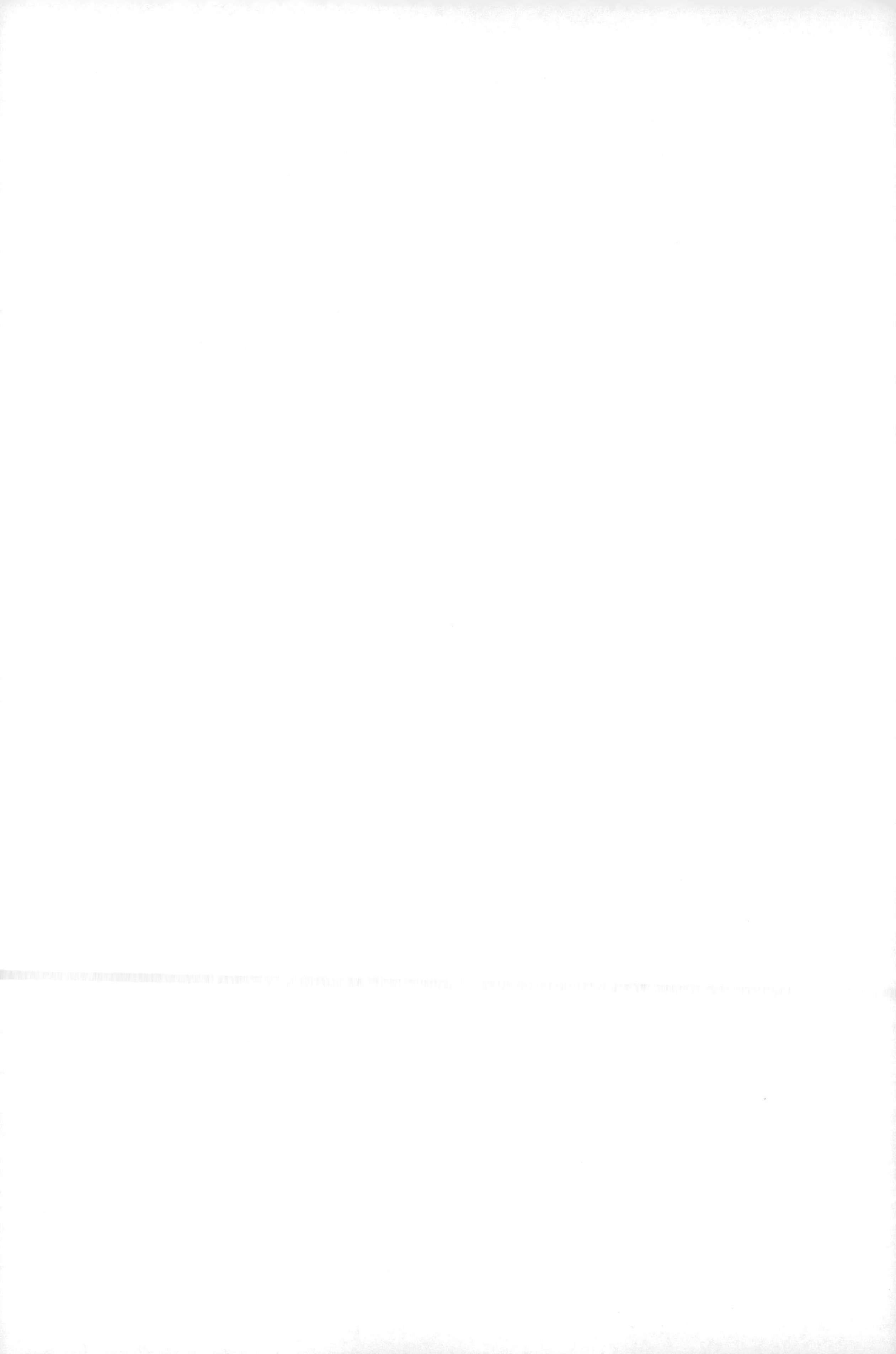

7 Hand-Assisted Laparoscopic Splenectomy

Hua Zhang, Yichao Wang, and Bing Peng

7.1 Background

Since Delaitre et al. [1] completed the first laparoscopic splenectomy since 1991 in the world, laparoscopic splenectomy has become the most common laparoscopic solid organ operation and gradually become the gold standard treatment of some spleen diseases [2–4].

However, laparoscopic splenectomy is more difficult than traditional open splenectomy, because it requires a good technical basis for laparoscopic surgery and a relatively long learning curve. Complete laparoscopic splenectomy lacks the tactile sensation and flexibility of direct contact with human hands. During the operation, the spleen and the splenic blood vessels are easily torn, resulting in intraoperative bleeding, which affects the surgical field of vision and even endangers the patient's life. Moreover, it is relatively difficult to control the bleeding under laparoscopy. In addition, for some huge spleen such as liver cirrhosis patients with portal hypertension patients, the operation space is small, and the quality of spleen is brittle, fragile, and easy bleeding; intraoperative traction or exposal is difficult; totally laparoscopic splenectomy is at high risk [3]. In order to overcome the above difficulties, hand-assisted laparoscopic splenectomy has gradually emerged combining the advantages of minimally invasive laparoscopic surgery and open surgery, and it has become an alternative for beginners in laparoscopic splenectomy principle.

Compared with the total laparoscopic splenectomy, hand-assisted laparoscopic splenectomy (HALS) is different in that the auxiliary hole is an incision about 7 cm long, a hand port is inserted into the abdominal cavity (as shown in Fig. 7.1), and the left hand can assist operation by touching the spleen directly to detect small lesions, to assist in drawing and showing, and to reduce bleeding, thus greatly reducing the operation difficulty [5].

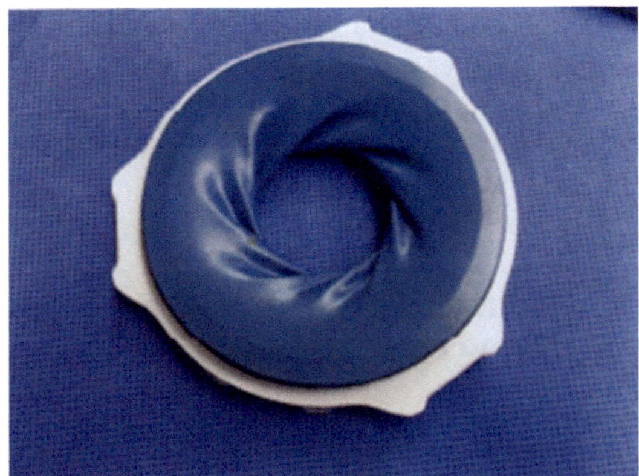

Fig. 7.1 Hand port

H. Zhang · Y. Wang · B. Peng (✉)
West China Hospital, Sichuan University, Chengdu, China

B. Peng (ed.), *Laparoscopic Surgery of the Spleen*, https://doi.org/10.1007/978-981-16-1216-9_7

7.2 Indications and Contraindications

7.2.1 Indications

The surgical indications of hand-assisted laparoscopic splenectomy are the same as those of open surgery [6], specifically including:

1. Splenomegaly caused by blood system diseases, such as thalassemia and hemolytic anemia
2. Secondary hypersplenism, such as cirrhotic portal hypertension with hypersplenism [7, 8]
3. Splenic malignant tumor, such as lymphoma and lymphatic sarcoma

7.2.2 Contraindications

Contraindications to hand-assisted laparoscopic splenectomy can be divided into absolute contraindications and relative contraindications [6].

1. Absolute contraindications include ① patients having difficulty in correcting coagulation disorders; ②patients with heart, lung, and other important organs functional insufficiency and without tolerance to general anesthesia surgery.
2. Relative contraindications include ① obese patients (BMI > 40) [9, 10]; ② patients with middle and third trimester pregnancy; ③ patients after splenic artery embolization [11–13] and shock due to traumatic splenic rupture and without improvement in hemodynamic index after correction [14].

7.3 Preoperative Assessment and Preparation

7.3.1 Physical Examination

Preoperative rigorous physical examination can preliminarily assess the size and boundary of the spleen, which is helpful for the selection of surgical methods and the distribution of preoperative puncture holes.

7.3.2 Assessment and Preparation of the Patients

Routine examination of the patient includes electrocardiogram, chest radiograph, blood routine, coagulation function, and liver and kidney function. For patients with abnormal coagulation function and poor liver function, surgical treatment should be performed after correction of coagulation function and liver or kidney function. However, for elderly patients (over 70 years old), preoperative echocardiography, pulmonary function testing, coronary artery CT, and other examinations should be selected according to the situation. Preoperative diseases such as hypertension and diabetes should be actively corrected before surgical treatment.

7.3.3 Imaging Examination

Patients with traumatic splenic rupture should be routinely assessed for the presence of other organ injuries by routine enhanced CT scan of the entire abdomen to fully identify the size and boundary of the spleen.

Based on the above assessment and preparation, the surgical methods and the distribution of Trocars are determined to greatly reduce the incidence of intraoperative and postoperative complications.

7.4 Surgical Procedures

7.4.1 Surgical Position and Surgeon Position

The surgical position and surgeon position are the same as those stated in Chap. 5 "Laparoscopic Splenectomy."

7.4.2 Main Steps

1. Make a 7 cm incision under the xiphoid process, enter the abdomen under direct vision, and place a hand port.
2. According to the size of the spleen and under the guidance of the left hand, a 10 mm incision in the umbilical cord or the lower right part of the umbilical cord is made, the pneumoperitoneum needle is inserted to establish the pneumoperitoneum, set the pneumoperitoneum pressure to 12–15 mmHg, and insert the puncture sheath (Trocar) and laparoscopic lens to explore the abdominal cavity.
3. Patients take the head high, foot low, and right oblique position. Under direct vision, in the corresponding position of the left clavicular line and the left axillary front line, a 12 mm incision and a 5 mm incision are made, and the puncture sheath is inserted.
4. Pull open the ligaments of the spleen and stomach with left hand and tow them by the assistant to maintain a certain tension (as shown in Fig. 7.2); break them with the ultrasonic scalpel or LigaSure, and reach up to the upper pole of the spleen and the splenic ligament (as shown in Fig. 7.3), and fully dissociate the upper pole of the spleen; pull up the lower pole of the spleen with left hand and pull the ligaments of the spleen and colon by the assistant (as shown in Fig. 7.4), and detach them with an ultrasonic scalpel; then, flip the spleen from the outside to the inside by the master operator with his left hand and dissociate the splenorenal ligament (as shown in Fig. 7.5).
5. Detach the splenic pedicle with Endo-GIA stapler (as shown in Fig. 7.6). The master operator separates the surrounding tissues of the splenic pedicle with the left thumb and

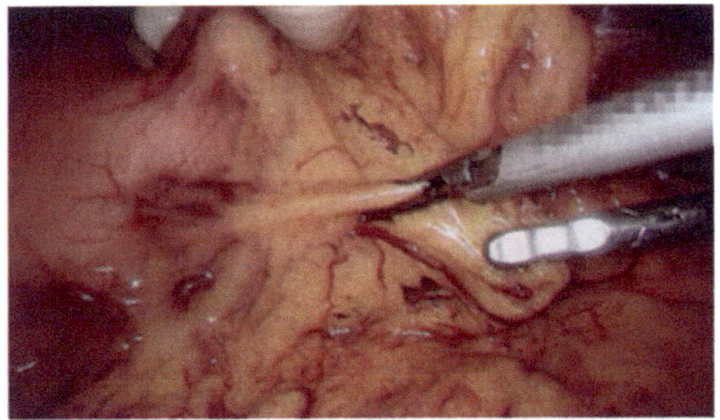

Fig. 7.2 Detachment of gastrosplenic ligament

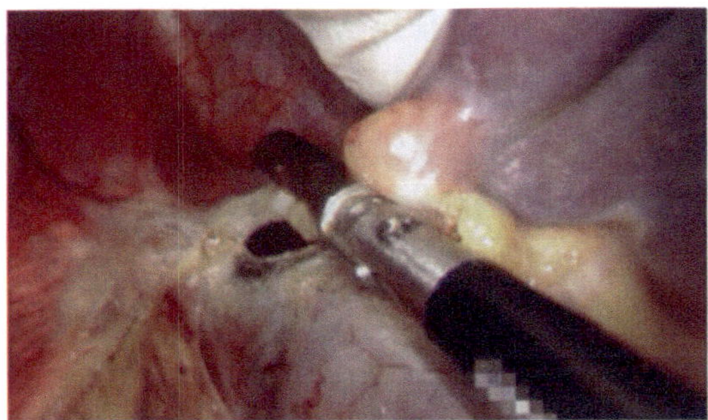

Fig. 7.3 Detachment of splenophrenic ligament

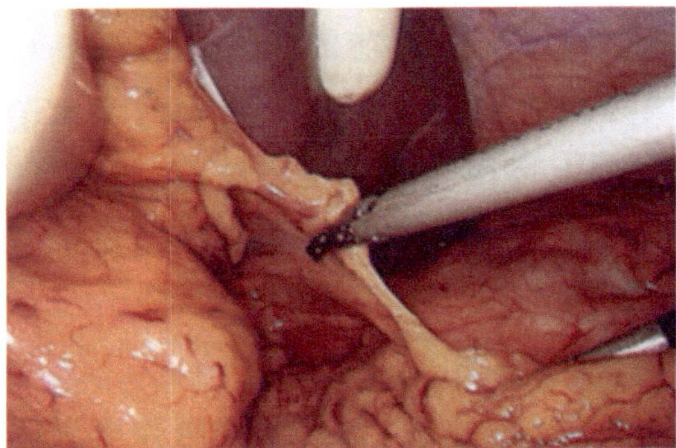

Fig. 7.4 Detachment of splenocolic ligament

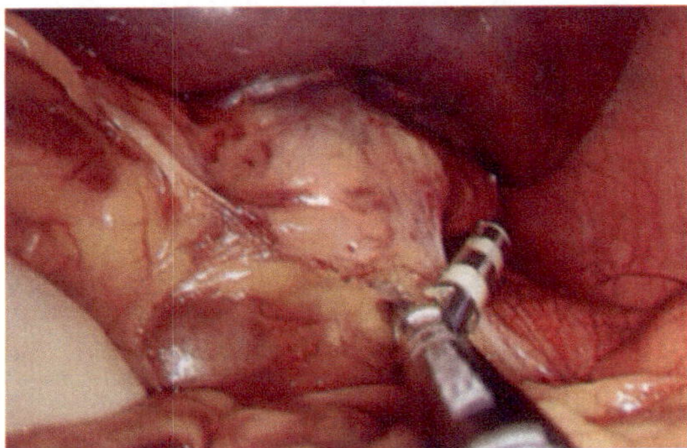

Fig. 7.5 Detachment of lienorenal ligament

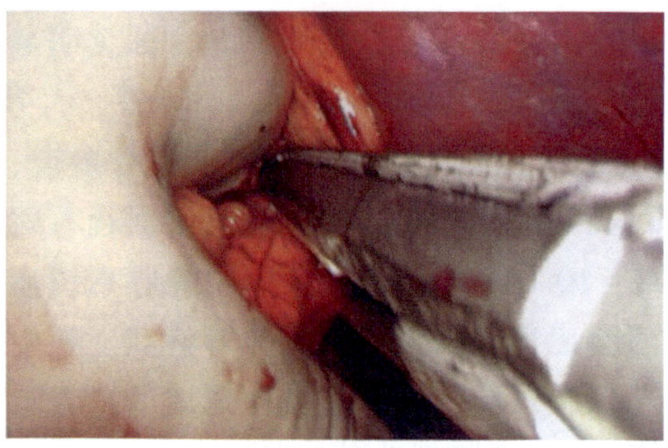

Fig. 7.6 Detachment of splenic pedicle with Endo-GIA stapler

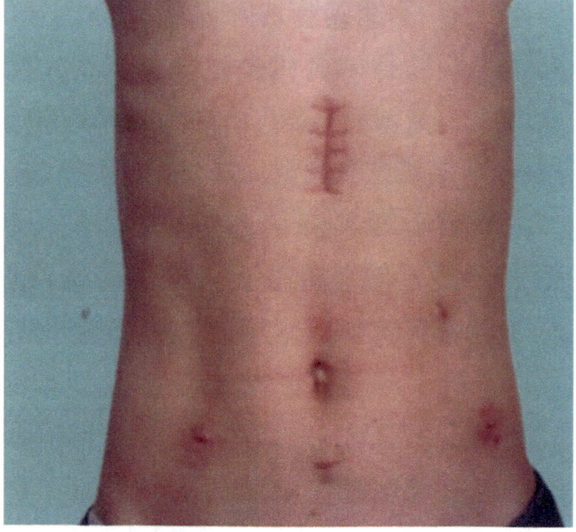

Fig. 7.7 Postoperative incision

index finger via the Toldt's fusion fascia, holds the splenic pedicle with left hand, and detaches it with a stapler. For the surgical wound hemostasis, take out of the spleen, place an orthopedic drainage tube in the splenic fossae, and close the abdominal incision (as shown in Fig. 7.7).

7.5 Key Surgical Techniques

The key operation steps and techniques are similar to those of laparoscopic splenectomy (for any information, refer to the related sections of Laparoscopic Splenectomy). Their difference lies in that, in case of splenic portal blood vessel injury or splenic bleeding, in order to prevent massive bleeding, the master operator can use the left thumb and index finger to clamp the splenic pedicle for temporary hemostasis or carry out blunt separation of the anterior and posterior splenic pedicle and use the Endo-GIA stapler to break the splenic pedicle for hemostasis. In this way, the incidence of intraoperative bleeding and conversion to open surgery can be effectively reduced.

7.6 Special Intraoperative Circumstances and Handling Skills

7.6.1 Bleeding

In case of bleeding during the operation, in order to prevent massive bleeding, the bleeding should not be stopped by blind clamp; instead, the master operator can use the left thumb and index finger to clamp the splenic pedicle for temporary hemostasis or carry out blunt separation of the anterior and posterior splenic pedicle and use the Endo-GIA stapler to break the splenic pedicle for hemostasis.

7.6.2 Peripheral Organ Injury

For the injury of gastric fundus, diaphragm, or prerenal fascia, suture repair can be performed; for the damage of the pancreatic tail, suture and ligation can be used to prevent pancreatic fistula. The drainage tube is routinely placed at the splenic fossa after the operation to monitor bleeding and pancreatic fistula.

7.7 Postoperative Management and Prevention and Treatment of Complications

7.7.1 Postoperative Management

For the key points of postoperative management, please refer to the related section in Chap. 5 "Laparoscopic Splenectomy."

7.7.2 Prevention and Treatment of Postoperative Complications

1. The common postoperative complications of hand-assisted laparoscopic splenectomy include bleeding, seroperitoneum, abscess formation, adjacent organ injury, and pulmonary infection. For the prevention and treatment, please refer to the related section in Chap. 5 "Laparoscopic Splenectomy."
2. Pancreatic fistula

   Pancreatic fistula is related to pancreatic injury and is a common complication in case of injury to tail of pancreas after detachment of splenic hilum distal pancreatectomy with Endo-GIA stapler [15]. Compared with laparoscopic splenectomy, hand-assisted laparoscopic splenectomy has the advantage that the master operator can use the left thumb and index finger to carry out blunt separation of the tail of pancreas and splenic hilum, so as to reduce the injury to tail of pancreas and the incidence of pancreatic fistula. In our center, we monitor the blood routine, biochemical complete set, coagulation, serum, and drainage fluid amylase on POD 1, POD 3, and POD 5. If pancreatic fistula infection occurs, somatostatin and anti-infection treatment should be given, and the drainage shall be kept normal with drainage tube. Color ultrasound examination of the abdominal cavity is performed when the abdominal drainage fluid is less than 5 mL/day or the content of amylase in drainage fluid is normal to determine whether the drainage tube could be extracted.
3. Portal vein thrombosis

   After splenectomy, the broken end of the splenic vein is the blind end, and changes in hemodynamics make it easy to form thrombosis. The incidence of splenic vein thrombosis after splenectomy can be as high as 20–55% [16], and sometimes splenic vein thrombosis can involve the portal vein, resulting in abnormal liver function, with an incidence of 6.3–10.0% [17]. For patients with postoperative portal vein thrombosis, most of them have no obvious clinical symptoms, and a small number of patients will have abdominal discomfort, low fever, and other symptoms. Our center routinely reviewed color Doppler ultrasound of portal vein system in patients with laparoscopic splenectomy 1 week after surgery and gave low-molecular-weight heparin anticoagulation treatment to patients with thrombosis. Previous studies have confirmed that after 10 days of anticoagulant treatment, the re-dredged rate of thrombus can reach 90% [18].

7.8 Hot Topics and Future Prospects

7.8.1 Advantages of HALS

Since the mid-1990s, hand-assisted instruments have appeared in the field of laparoscopic surgery [19–21], and HALS has been gradually developed in clinical practice.

Hand-assisted laparoscopic surgery is a new and improved minimally invasive surgery, which has the advantages of minimally invasive laparoscopic surgery and open surgery. In HALS surgery, the left hand of the surgeons can put into the abdominal cavity and directly contact the spleen through the special chiral auxiliary equipment to retain the advantage of the precise tactile feedback by the operator with fingers and facilitate intraoperative diagnosis of pathological changes. In addition, the left hand can serve as a retractor, so as to help to pull ligament around spleen to expose and separate it.

During the operation, the left hand can directly contact the spleen or the spleen pedicle. When there is damaged bleeding during the operation, the left hand can compress the spleen or the spleen pedicle to control the bleeding and expose the bleeding points, so as to facilitate the hemostasis and improve the safety of the operation. The left hand can be used to completely push away the pancreatic tail to avoid damaging it when the splenic pedicle is severed with the straight cutting closure device, and the straight cutting closure device can be guided to place the splenic pedicle completely into the staple cartridge to ensure the complete separation of the splenic pedicle. Moreover, the resected surgical specimens can be put into the specimen bag and removed directly by hand with the aid of incision, which can shorten the time of spleen collection and operation, at the same time, avoiding the risk of specimen bag rupture and spleen implantation [22]. HALS surgery has a mild impact on the body's inflammatory response to trauma and immune function and a relatively small impact on the body's stress response, so it has the advantage of minimally invasive surgery [23]. HALS as a kind of modified laparoscopic surgery, minimally invasive surgery, and the advantage of open operation, compared with the total laparoscopic splenectomy, reduces the difficulty of the procedure, shortens the operation time, reduces the rate of transfer laparotomy, reduces the intraoperative blood loss, and improves the operation safety [24–26]; it has built a bridge between laparoscopic splenectomy and open splenectomy for beginners. At the same time, it provides a new minimally invasive surgical method for some patients who have difficulty in complete laparoscopic splenectomy.

7.8.2 Disadvantages of HALS

Since the left hand enters the abdominal cavity, the operation space in the abdominal cavity is further reduced, which will seriously affect the surgical field of vision and hinder the flexibility of operation. In addition, with the extension of the operation time, the hand of the surgeon will appear ischemia, swelling, numbness, and paresthesia, which will affect the smooth operation and cause occupational injuries to the hand of the surgeon.

7.8.3 Future Prospects

As abovementioned, HALS has two disadvantages, i.e., the reduced operation space caused by the left hand of the surgeon and the press of the left hand caused by the hand-assisted instrument. Therefore, a robot arm should be invented to simulate the function of the left hand of the surgeon and the tactile feedback of the instrument, so as to avoid the reduced operation space and the damaging press. HALS, as a modified laparoscopic surgery, can serve as a transition surgery from open splenectomy to complete laparoscopic splenectomy, which will help the learner to smoothly go through the learning curve period. We believe the surgery will have more indications with the development of technology and instruments and be further extended to the operations of such organs as liver, cholecyst and pancreas. Moreover, the operation results will be better accepted by both the surgeon and the patient.

References

1. Delaitre B, Maignien B. Splenectomy by the laparoscopic approach. Report of a case. Presse Med. 1992;20(44):2263.
2. Wang YB. Research progress of laparoscopic splenectomy. J Modern Med Health. 2017;33(10):1494–7.
3. Zhu JF, Chen J, Zhang HY, et al. Hand-assisted laparoscopic splenectomy. Proc 2003 Natl Acad Conf Adv Minim Invasive Surg. 2003;2003:122–4.
4. Habermalz B, Sauerland S, Decker G, et al. Laparoscopic splenectomy: the clinical practice guidelines of the European Association for Endoscopic Surgery (EAES). Sug Endosc. 2008;22(4):821–48.
5. Liu Y, Wang H, Duan SB. Laparoscopic-assisted versus open splenectomy: a systematic review of domestic studies. Chinese J Gen Surg. 2013;22(6):756–61.
6. Smith L, Luna G, Mera AR, et al. Laparoscopic splenectomy for treatment of splenomegaly. Am J Surg. 2004;187(5):618–20.
7. Kawanaka H, Akahoshi T, Kinjo N, et al. Technical standardization of laparoscopic splenectomy harmonized with handassisted laparoscopic surgery for patients with liver cirrhosis and hypersplenism. Hepatobil Pancreat Surg. 2009;16(6):749–57.
8. Chen SF, Li XM, Chen HM. Comparison of hand-assisted laparoscopic splenectomy plus porta-agygous devascularization and open splenectomy. J Nanchang Univ (Med Sci). 2011;48(3):40–2.
9. Dominguez EP, Choi YU, Scott BG, et al. Impact of morbid obesity on outcome of laparoscopic splenectomy. Surg Endosc. 2007;21(3):422–6.
10. Schlachta CM, Poulin EC, Mamazza J. Laparoscopic splenectomy for hematologic malignancies. Surg Endosc. 1999;13(9):865–8.
11. Cao XF, Liu QH. Effect of splenic artery embolization on reoperation of recurrent hypersplenism. Chin J Gen Practition. 2012;11(12):943–4.

12. Zheng GQ, Liang JR, Zhang YZ, et al. Three cases of splenectomy after splenic artery embolization. J Pract Med. 2012;28(20):3497–8.
13. Lv JL, Li XP, Yang SW, et al. Laparoscopic splenectomy and pericardial devascularization for splenomegaly: a report of 15 cases. Chinese J Minim Invas Surg. 2013;13(5):406.
14. Wang GY, Jiang C. Development and practice of laparoscopic splenectomy. Chinese J Hepat Surg (Electron Ed). 2017;6(4):241–4.
15. Bie P, Chen J. Laparoscopic splenectomy. Chinese J Hepat Surg (Electron Ed). 2015;3:142–5.
16. Bhandarkar DS, Katara AN, Mittal G, et al. Prevention and management of complications of laparoscopic splenectomy. Indian J Surg. 2011;73(5):327–30.
17. Hassan AM, AI-Fallouji MA, Ouf TI, et al. Portal vein thrombosis following splenectomy. Br J Surg. 2000;87(3):362–73.
18. van't Reit M, Burger J, Van Muiswinkel J, et al. Diagnosis and treatment of portal vein thrombosis following splenectomy. Br J Surg. 2000;87(9):1229–33.
19. Krauth MT, Lechner K, Neugebauer EA, et al. The postoperative splenic/portal vein thrombosis after splenectomy and its prevention-an unresolved issue. Haematologica. 2008;93(8):1227–32.
20. Romano F, Caprotti R, Conti M, et al. Thrombosis of the splenoportal axis after splenectomy. Langenbeck's Arch Surg. 2006;391(5):483–8.
21. Demetrius E, Litwin AD, Jacek J, et al. Hand-assisted laparoscopic surgery (HALS) with the hand port system initial experience with 68 patients. Ann Surg. 2000;231(5):715–23.
22. Sang JY, He JY. Clinical comparative study of hand-assisted laparoscopic and open splenectomy and pericardial devascularization. J Laparosc Surg. 2013;12(10):758–60.
23. Feng ZR, He XW, Liao K. Effect of hand-assistant laparoscopic splenectomy plus pericardial devascularization and open surgery on immune system and wound responses. China J Endosc. 2003;9(7):39–41.
24. Moreno SC, Noguera JF, Herrero ML, et al. Single incision laparoscopic surgery. Cir Esp. 2010;88(1):12–7.
25. Barbaros U, Dinccag A, Sumer A, et al. Prospective randomized comparison of clinical results between hand-assisted laparoscopic and open splenectomies. Surg Endosc. 2010;24:25–32.
26. Gamme G, Birch DW, Karmali S. Minimally invasive splenectomy: an update and review. Can J Surg. 2013;56(4):280–5.

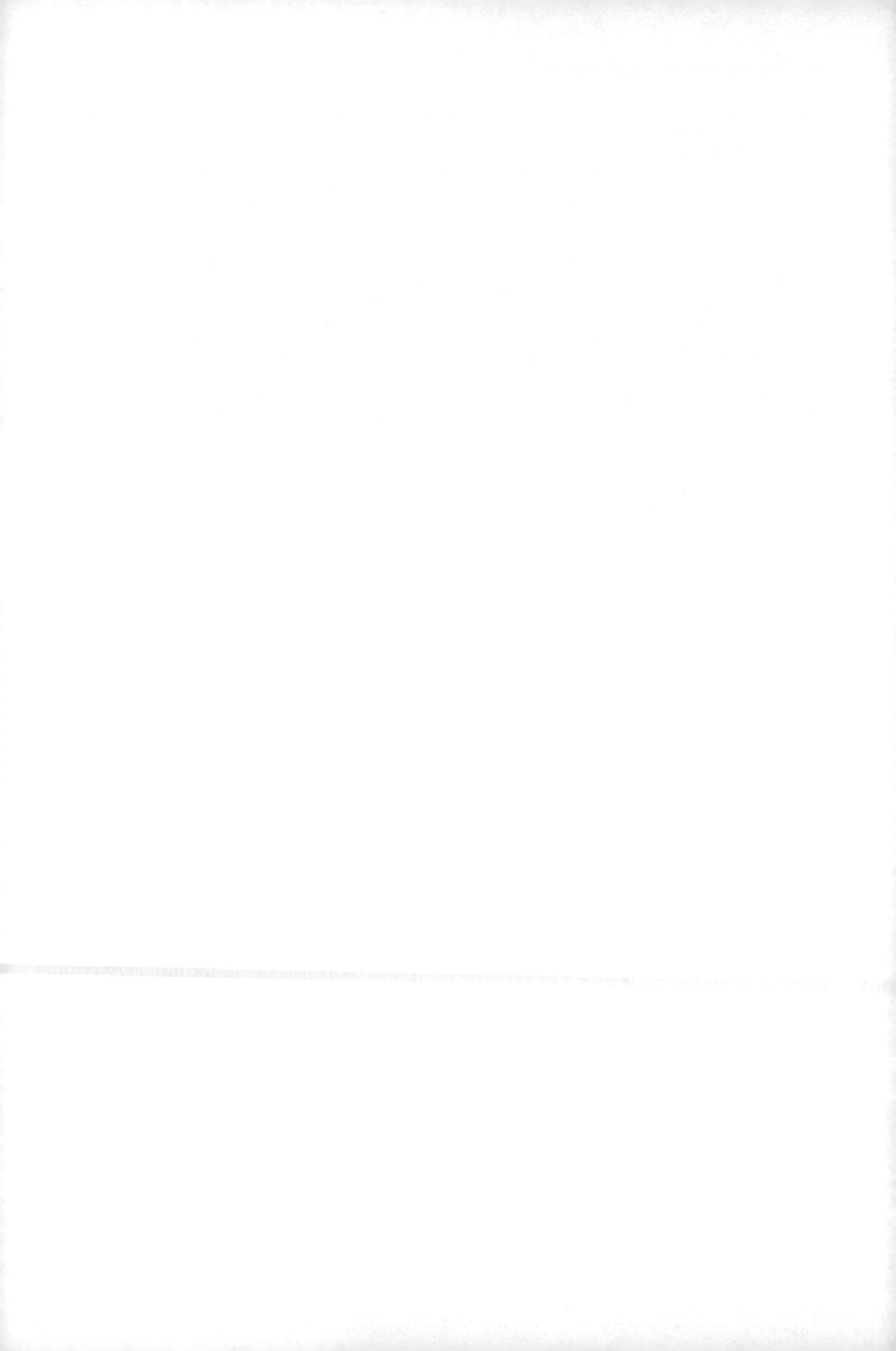

8 Laparoscopic Partial Splenectomy

Yongbin Li, Xin Wang, Junfeng Wang, Ke Chen, and Bing Peng

8.1 Background

Spleen is a critical immune organ with anti-infection and immune functions. Overwhelming post-splenectomy infection (OPSI) is a deadly infection due to weakened immunity after splenectomy, and the pathogenic bacteria mainly include *Streptococcus pneumoniae*, *Haemophilus influenzae* type B, and *Neisseria meningitidis*. A study found that the morbidity of OPSI in patients after splenectomy is 5% (including short-term and long-term morbidity), and the mortality is 200 times higher than normal people [1]. Another study published in Lancet found that 33% patients after splenectomy would receive hospitalization treatment in 10 years due to infection of various reasons [2]. Furthermore, many long-term complications of splenectomy have been reported as follows: pulmonary arterial hypertension, atherosclerosis, coronary heart disease, and tumor [3, 4]. Meanwhile, secondary thrombocytosis and hemodynamic changes after splenectomy would increase the risk of thrombosis in splenic vein, portal vein, and mesenteric vein [5]. In general, an increasing number of surgeons have attached importance to reserve spleen function and various ways to preserve the spleen functions have been found.

One way to preserve the spleen functions is splenic autotransplantation developed in the 1980s. With the splenic autotransplantation method, the remnant healthy spleen tissue after spleen removal is transplanted into omentum majus for function preservation. However, many studies proved that the transplanted spleen is hard to realize functional compensation after surgery due to lack of natural blood supply [2, 6]. Another way is partial splenic embolization (PSE). With the partial splenic embolization method, partial spleen vessels are blocked to cause ischemic infarction of corresponding spleen parenchyma, so it can be used in patients with hypersplenism secondary to portal hypertension, hereditary spherocytosis, and traumatic splenic rupture [7]. Nevertheless, this way only achieves "similar resection" that aseptic necrosis of corresponding spleen parts is realized through selective blocking of partial spleen vessels, but fails to eradicate the root cause of spleen disease. Moreover, patients may take risks of hyperpyrexia, abdominal pain, and abscess formation after surgery. So the application of PSE is limited in the treatment of splenic surgical diseases. Compared with the two ways above, partial splenectomy can not only preserve the spleen functions but also prevent postoperative ischemic spleen infarction after operation by selective devascularization of spleen vessels and

Y. Li · X. Wang · K. Chen · B. Peng (✉)
West China Hospital, Sichuan University, Chengdu, China

J. Wang
The First People's Hospital of Yunnan Province, Kunming, China

B. Peng (ed.), *Laparoscopic Surgery of the Spleen*, https://doi.org/10.1007/978-981-16-1216-9_8

partial excision of the spleen. The method was found by Prof. Morgenstern [8] in the 1980s, and it has been widely used in various splenic surgical diseases, including splenic neoplasia, spleen abscess, and hematological system diseases mentioned above.

Laparoscopic splenectomy (LS) is currently widely used in clinic [9]. However, laparoscopic partial splenectomy (LPS) requires more skillful operation technique than LS, so that to date there is no evidence to support broad clinical applications of LPS. In this chapter, we will share the experience and techniques of our clinical center in LPS and will also discuss relative reports from others at home and overseas to demonstrate the method more comprehensively.

8.2 Indications and Contraindications

8.2.1 Indications

8.2.1.1 Splenic Neoplasia

Splenic neoplasia is located in the upper or lower pole of spleen. Large neoplasia should be treated with LPS only after being assessed by imaging examination to determine that the residue spleen volume is bigger than 25% (capable of compensating the spleen functions) of full spleen volume [2]. The pathologic diagnosis includes nonparasitic cysts, hemangioma, and lymphangioma.

8.2.1.2 Traumatic Rupture of the Spleen

Most of traumatic ruptures of the spleen can be treated with good result by conservative treatment or interventional embolization [10]. Surgery is only suitable for patients with bad results from above treatment. Due to long operation time, our center only includes patients with stable hemodynamics, but without other organ injury and vessel condition to receive interventional embolization.

8.2.2 Contraindications

For patients with traumatic rupture of the spleen, unstable signs of life or massive hemorrhage during operation are the primary contraindications of LPS. Other contraindications include large neoplasia with the remnant spleen less than 25% after partial splenectomy, neoplasia relative to parasites with risk of intraoperative rupture and dissemination, and severe dense adhesion around hilum of spleen that is hard to separate.

8.3 Preoperative Assessment and Preparation

8.3.1 Basic Assessment of Patient

Basic assessment includes ECG (electrocardiogram), chest radiography, blood routine, coagulation function, hepatic and renal function, and nutrition condition. Systematic assessments should be applied to elder patients (older than 70 years), including echocardiography, pulmonary function test, and coronary computed tomography angioplasty. Hypertension and diabetes should be controlled before operation. Patients with traumatic rupture of the spleen should be assessed by hemodynamic monitoring (according to definitions in Advanced Life Support (Ninth Edition), unstable hemodynamic condition means blood press less than 90 mmHg and heart rate faster than 120 beats/min, accompanied with peripheral circulation disturbance, consciousness change and accelerated breathing).

8.3.2 Radiography Assessment

For patients with splenic neoplasia, upper abdomen computed tomography angiography should be routinely conducted to comprehend focus characteristics such as benign or malignant, size, location, and vessel, and other software should also be used to measure the neoplasia's volume. For patients with traumatic rupture of the spleen, head chest abdomen contrast-enhanced CT should be routinely conducted to assess other organs injury, the type of spleen injury (hematoma, tear, and breakage), and location.

We can judge patients through assessment and preparation as mentioned above whether patients are fit for LPS and decrease incidence of intraoperative and postoperative complications through adjusting patients' body condition before operation.

8.3.3 Preoperative Preparation

Preoperative preparation should be made as described in Chap. 5 (preoperative preparation of laparoscopic splenectomy). Meanwhile, red cell suspension and plasma should be prepared for use.

8.4 Surgical Procedures

Currently there are two operation methods for LPS: routine LPS and selective splenic pedicle occlusion (SSPO). In routine LPS, the surgeon dissects branch vessels of the splenic hilum without blocking splenic artery, and this method is applied for patients with simple anatomy of splenic hilum blood vessels. In SSPO, the splenic artery will be pre-blocked before dissection, and this method is applied for patients with complicated anatomy of splenic hilum blood vessels, hard to reserve spleen, traumatic rupture of spleen, and high risk of hemorrhage during operation.

8.4.1 Surgical Position and Surgeon Position

Both methods are performed with supine elevated position, leaning to the right by 30–45 degrees. Pneumoperitoneum pressure is 13 mmHg with 10 mm trocar at the periumbilicus as observation hole, 5 mm trocar below the xiphoid as the assistant hole, 12 mm trocar at left mid-clavicular line below the costal margin as the main operation hole, and 5 mm trocar at left anterior axillary line below the costal margin as the assistant operation hole (Fig. 8.1).

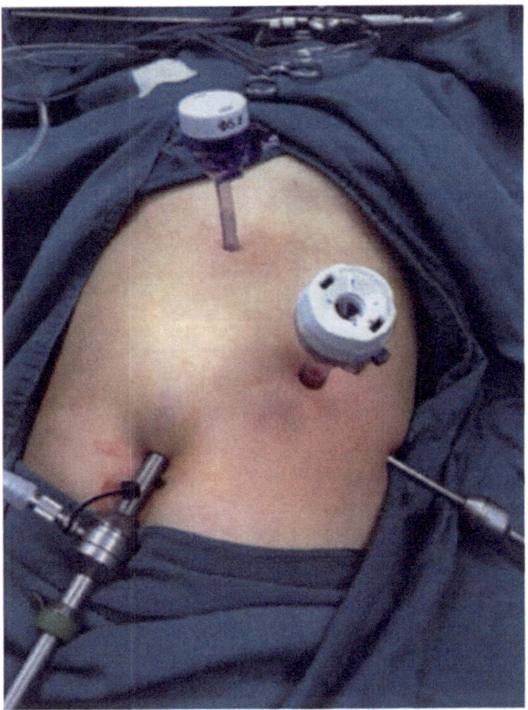

Fig. 8.1 Trocar placement

8.4.2 Main Steps

8.4.2.1 Routine LPS

1. Dissociating spleen: open the spleen gastric ligament with ultrasound scalpel, and dissociate the ligament around the spleen to be dissected. If the location of lesion is at the inferior pole of spleen, sufficiently dissociate the inferior splenic ligaments, including lower parts of splenocolic ligament, splenorenal ligament, phrenicocolic ligament, and gastrosplenic ligament, but reserving the splenophrenic ligament and short gastric vessel (Fig. 8.2). If the location of lesion is at the superior pole of spleen, sufficiently dissociate the upper parts of splenophrenic ligament, gastrosplenic ligament, and splenorenal ligament.
2. Dissecting spleen portal vessel: dissect branch of spleen veins and artery around the lesion. Ligate and disconnect these vessels and

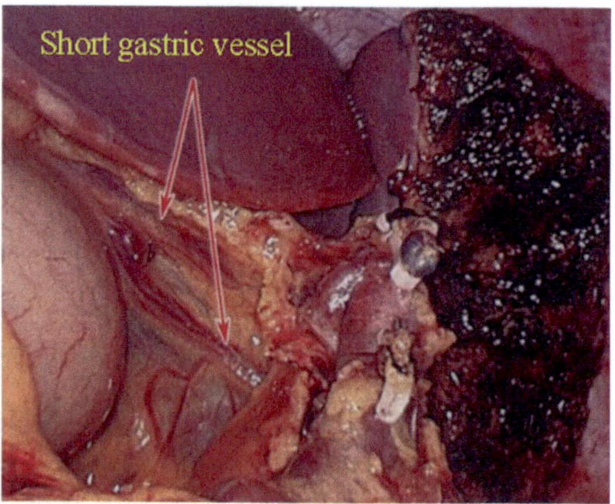

Fig. 8.2 Reserving the short gastric vessel

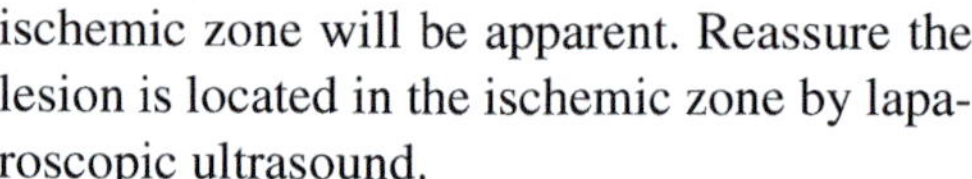

ischemic zone will be apparent. Reassure the lesion is located in the ischemic zone by laparoscopic ultrasound.

3. Cutting off spleen: cut off spleen in the ischemic zone around 0.5–1 cm to the ischemic line with an ultrasound scalpel little by little from front to back. Coagulate in case of active bleeding. Completely resect the lesion.
4. Hemostasis of spleen section and fixation of rest spleen: coagulate the section by unipolar or bipolar electrocautery. Fix the rest of spleen on the lateral abdominal wall or connective tissue of spleen by vascular line if the spleen moves in a large range. Take out specimen by the peri-umbilicus incision. Put a drainage tube at spleen fossa. The surgery is completed.

8.4.2.2 Selective Splenic Pedicle Occlusion

1. Dissociating spleen: as described above, open spleen gastric ligament and dissociate ligaments around the spleen to be dissected.
2. Selective splenic pedicle occlusion: open retroperitoneum at upper pancreas and find the splenic artery trunk, and block the trunk by splenic pedicle blocking clamp. It can be used for patients with traumatic splenic rupture, complex branch vessels, and difficult anatomy (Fig. 8.3).

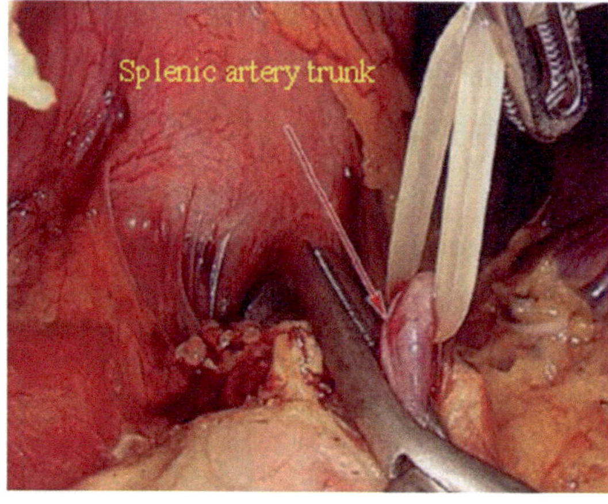

Fig. 8.3 Blocking the splenic artery

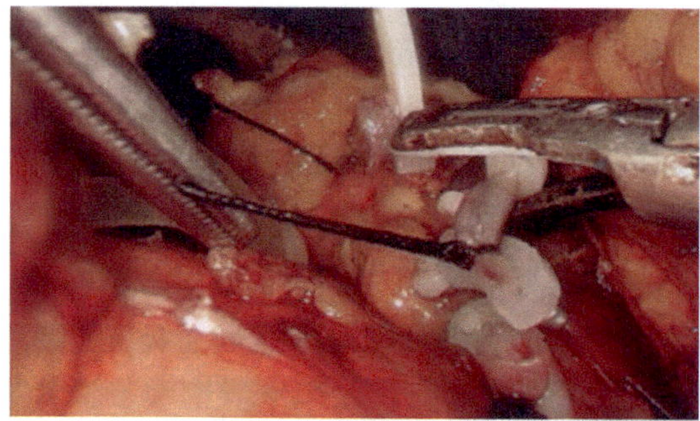

Fig. 8.4 Dissecting branch vessel

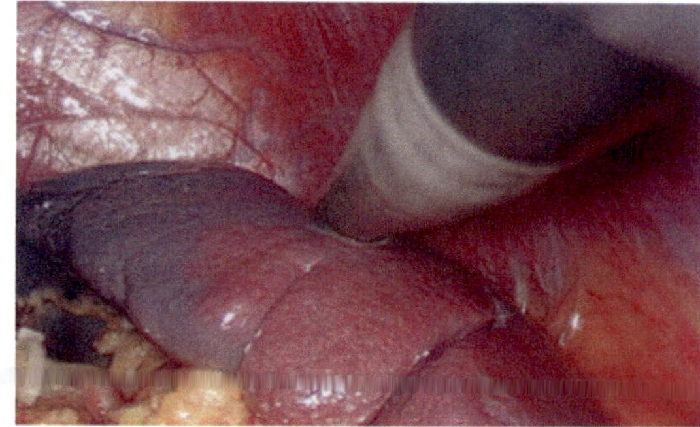

Fig. 8.5 Reassuring the resection area by laparoscopic ultrasound

3. Dissecting branch vessels and dissociating the spleen: as described above, disconnect the splenic artery and branch of splenic veins of the lesion (Fig. 8.4). Reassure the resection area by laparoscopic ultrasound (Fig. 8.5).

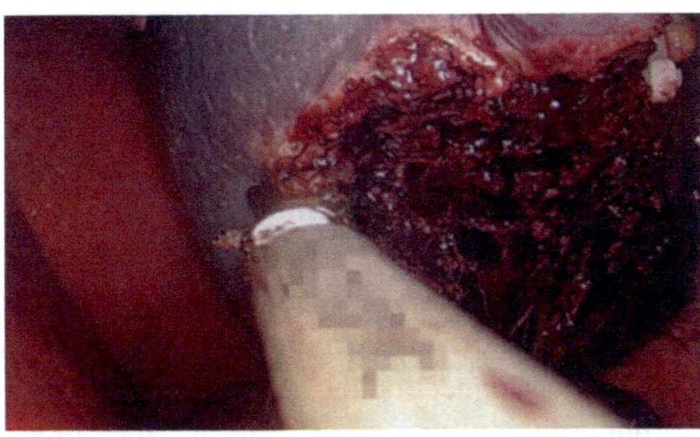

Fig. 8.6 Disconnecting the spleen with an ultrasound scalpel

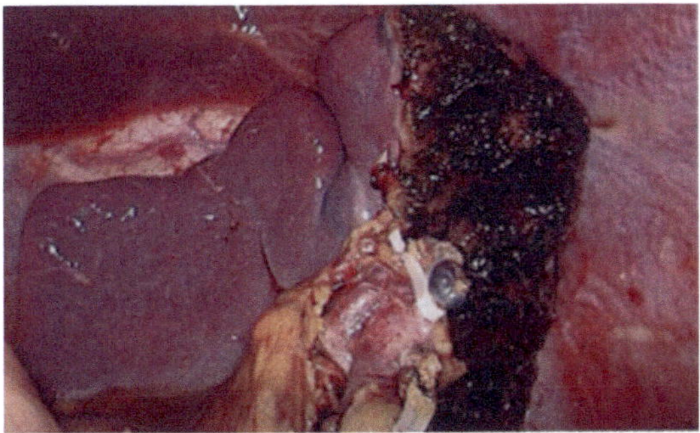

Fig. 8.7 Hemostasis of spleen section

Disconnect the spleen to the ischemic line with an ultrasound scalpel (Fig. 8.6).

4. Ending the blocking and hemostasis of spleen section: coagulate the section by unipolar or bipolar electrocautery (Fig. 8.7). Release the splenic pedicle blocking clamp, and reassure no bleeding in section. Take out specimen and put a drainage tube at spleen fossa. The surgery is completed.

8.5 Key Surgical Techniques

8.5.1 Dissection of Spleen Vessels

It is the most important step in laparoscopic partial splenectomy. Preoperative assessment of the distribution pattern of spleen vessels can guide the operation. Face the non-working tip of ultrasound scalpel to the spleen vessels to avoid direct thermal damage in the procedure of dissecting the second spleen vessels. Dissect the superficial splenic artery to expose the deeper splenic vein, and then disconnect splenic vein. When patients have complex branch vessels, first block the trunk and then dissect the spleen vessels.

8.5.2 Intraoperative Location of Splenic Space-Occupying Lesions

It is easy to recognize superficial lesions in operation. For patients with deeper lesions or multi-lesions, laparoscopic ultrasound should be used to locate the lesions accurately to avoid omitting the lesions.

8.5.3 Hemostasis of Spleen Section

The options for stopping bleeding include monopolar coagulation scalpels, bipolar coagulation scalpels, and hectogram pliers. For hemostasis of spleen section, follow the order from top to bottom. In case of less bleeding, use monopolar coagulation scalpel; in case of massive bleeding, use bipolar coagulation scalpels and hectogram pliers. Intravenous drip of normal saline is helpful.

8.6 Special Intraoperative Circumstances and Handling Skills

8.6.1 Bleeding During the Dissection of Spleen Hilum

We use the primary splenic pedicle dissection way in laparoscopic splenectomy and thus will not dissect the secondary splenic pedicle. When it comes to laparoscopic partial splenectomy, we should dissect the secondary splenic pedicle. Bleeding during the dissection of spleen hilum is the common complication at the beginning of laparoscopic partial splenectomy, which is also the common reason for converting to open surgery or laparoscopic splenectomy. The usual reasons of bleeding are unfamiliarity with anatomy or thermal injury of vessels due to the false usage of ultrasound scalpel. Sometimes the bleeding comes from vessel injury when dissecting the splenic vessels or rupture of spleen. Vessel injury in small branches of splenic vessels or upper or lower parts of spleen results in less bleeding. Vessel injury in trunk of splenic vessels or splenic lobe often results in fast and massive bleeding.

1. Bleeding in distal vessels: The laparoscopic navigator cleans the camera shot immediately to keep the clear field of view when the shot is stained due to bleeding. The assistant presses the bleeding spot by an aspirator. The operator pulls the tissue around the omentum, dispose the bleeding spot, control the bleeding spot, and stop bleeding by Hem-o-lok, titanium clip, ultrasound scalpel, and LigaSure. Besides, it is also feasible to press the bleeding spot by gauze, aspirate the blood to dispose bleeding spot, and stop bleeding by clip or suture.
2. Bleeding in trunk or main branch splenic vein: Bleeding in the trunk is hard to control, and the blood will occupy the whole space of left upper abdomen. Operator and assistant can use the bleeding method mentioned above if they are familiar with laparoscopic operation. If the bleeding does not stop, stop it by gauze temporarily. Convert to open surgery immediately or put a hand-assistive device 7 cm under xiphoid. The operator controls spleen pedicle to stop bleeding by the left hand. After aspirating all blood, use a bulldog clamp to block splenic artery near-end, and operate to stop bleeding if the bleeding spot is at the far-end of branch of splenic artery. If the bleeding in the trunk of splenic artery or vein is hard to control, splenectomy is suggested. Therefore, we suggest using selective splenic pedicle occlusion in laparoscopic partial splenectomy. Find the splenic artery trunk at upper pancreas, and block the trunk by splenic pedicle blocking clamp, which could decrease the risk of massive bleeding in splenic artery and intraoperative bleeding.
3. Bleeding in splenic injury: The same as laparoscopic splenectomy in Chap. 5.

8.6.2 Adjacent Organ Injury

1. Diaphragm injury: It usually happens if the operator fails to recognize the diaphragm when disconnecting the spleen around the diaphragmatic surface. Repairing the injury needs the cooperation with anesthetist in the end of inhale. Conduct thoracic close drainage when necessary. Fill a piece of gauze under diaphragm intraoperatively to avoid diaphragm injury and thermal injury by the ultrasound scalpel.
2. Stomach injury: The same as laparoscopic splenectomy in Chap. 5.
3. Injury in the splenocolic area: The same as laparoscopic splenectomy in Chap. 5.
4. Pancreas injury: The same as laparoscopic splenectomy in Chap. 5.

8.7 Postoperative Management and Prevention and Treatment of Complications

8.7.1 Postoperative Management

The postoperative management of laparoscopic partial splenectomy follows the postoperative management in Chap. 5.

8.7.2 Prevention and Treatment of Postoperative Complications

1. Postoperative bleeding: The postoperative bleeding of laparoscopic partial splenectomy is associated with inadequate intraoperative hemostasis. It usually occurs in pancreas tail, short gastric vessel, and location of piercing sheath. The manifestation and diagnosis or treatment of bleeding is the same as laparo-

scopic splenectomy in Chap. 5. Especially for the main operative hole, according to our experience, the common practice is to suture the main operative hole by close observation and close peritoneum. Empty the air, rebuild the pneumoperitoneum after waiting for 10 min, and put in the laparoscope to observe. Pre-divide the splenic vessels before disconnecting spleen limiting in the ischemic zone. The bleeding in the section less happens, but thorough electrocoagulation of the splenic section is important for beginners.
2. Left subdiaphragmatic abscess and hydrops: The same as laparoscopic splenectomy in Chap. 5.
3. Portal vein thrombosis: Portal vein thrombosis is the common complication after laparoscopic splenectomy [11], which is related to air pressure, platelet elevation after splenectomy and portal vein hemodynamics change. Laparoscopic partial splenectomy reserves partial splenic function, but with rare platelet elevation after splenectomy and portal vein hemodynamics change and portal vein thrombosis. The diagnosis and treatment of portal vein thrombosis is the same as laparoscopic splenectomy in Chap. 5 with a high recanalization rate after treatment [12].

8.8 Hot Topics and Future Prospects

8.8.1 Theoretical Basis of Laparoscopic Partial Splenectomy

Laparoscopic partial splenectomy is based on deep research of anatomy and function of spleen. Liu and Poulin et al. [13, 14] found through spleen dissection that the spleen is similar to the liver in terms of lobe and segment distribution, i.e., with upper lobe and lower lobe and 3–5 segments, with independent blood supply and venous drainage system for each segment, but without vessel zone between segments. According to the location of spleen vessels, it can be divided into three kinds: dispersion (80% patients' splenic artery branch in 2.1–6 cm into spleen), middle (14% patients' splenic artery branch in 0.6–2 cm into spleen), and dense (6% patients' splenic artery branch close to hilus lienis). Splenic blood supply comes from splenic artery and arcus vasculosi of greater curvature. Blocking of these arteries will show the ischemia zone in the lobe or segment. Dissection in the ischemia zone can lessen bleeding. This research breaks the opinion that hemostasis after spleen section is hard. With the in-depth study on spleen function, it is found that spleen has the functions of immunity, anti-cancer, and decreasing morbidity in coronary heart disease and stroke. Kristinsson et al. [15] conducted a follow-up visit to 8149 veterans with laparoscopic splenectomy in 27 years. They found the morbidity of infection, cancer, coronary heart disease, and pulmonary embolism is increased compared with the control groups. This study again promoted the conduct of laparoscopic partial splenectomy.

8.8.2 Discussion on Indications of Laparoscopic Partial Splenectomy

The goal of laparoscopic partial splenectomy is to remove the lesion while reserving the splenic function. But the operation is limited by some indications. In Western countries, the incidence of hereditary spherocytosis is high and the patients usually have anemia because of hypersplenism, as well as anemia in different degree. Partial splenectomy can reserve splenic function and decrease the destruction of red blood cells. But there is no consensus on how much spleen can reserve its function, and some reports suggest that 10–25% is effective. Stoehr et al. [16, 17] from Germany believed that patients with hereditary spherocytosis should keep 10% of the spleen to reserve the immune and phagocytosis function. Di Sabatino and Uranues [18, 19] reported that at least 25% of the spleen could keep the splenic function. Meanwhile the rest spleen after laparoscopic partial splenectomy will be restricted by basic diseases. Patients with hereditary spherocytosis are affected by anemia and basic pathological change, and their spleen increases in tissues. However, for patients with splenic space-occupying lesions, the increase in spleen tissues is insignificant because of no stimulation from anemia and pathological change. Currently, it is believed that reserving 25% of the spleen is reasonable according to research. After splenectomy the rest volume of the spleen larger than 25% is an indication of patients with nonparasitic cyst, hamartoma, hemangioma, and metastatic tumors [18, 19]. For patients receiving selective operation, the rest volume should be calculated by three-dimensional reconstruction. For patients with severe adhesion, especially in hilus lienis, obesity, or intraoperative insufficient exposal, and with the rest volume of the spleen less than 25%, it is not recommended to receive the operation.

The treatment of traumatic splenic rupture is divided into two types: operative treatment or nonoperative treatment. Nonoperative treatment includes interventional therapy and conservative treatment. It is the standard treatment to patients with stable hemodynamics [20]. However, Brugere in France reported patients with stable hemodynamics treated by interventional therapy had 41% morbidity rates, including subdural hemorrhage, pleural effusion, infection, and splenic abscess [21]. Meanwhile, Moreno reported that patients with nonoperative treatment had 34% morbidity of abdominal pain and intra-abdominal infection and some patients needed operation to solve these complications [22]. Our previous study found that the postoperative morbidity of laparoscopic partial splenectomy was 7.5%, shown in hydrops. We disconnected spleen in the ischemic zone around 1 cm to the ischemic line with less intraoperative bleeding and decreasing the incidence of ischemia and splenic abscess [23]. The result is similar to the result of Balaphas et al. that 6.5% morbidity and similar kinds of complication [16]. So we suggest emergency laparoscopic partial splenectomy is an optional treatment to patients with stable hemodynamics without other organ injury. It is a minimally invasive operation to decrease postoperative morbidity while reserving the splenic function. But it should be conducted in experienced laparoscopic surgery centers.

8.8.3 Intraoperative Bleeding Control of Laparoscopic Partial Splenectomy

Our center has conducted this kind of surgery since 2011. Currently more than 60 cases of laparoscopic partial splenectomy have been accomplished. In clinical practice, we optimize flow of operation and propose selective splenic pedicle occlusion to decrease intraoperative bleeding to enhance the safety, especially to beginner operators and patients with complicated hilus lienis. Spleen is an organ with abundant blood supply, restricted by operation space, cooperation, and device operation skills. It is usually converted into open surgery or laparoscopic splenectomy when hemostasis occurs. So how to decrease or prevent hemostasis is the key of laparoscopic partial splenectomy. Selective splenic pedicle occlusion is important to patients who undergo laparoscopic partial splenectomy with traumatic splenic rupture and complex splenic vessels. First open retroperitoneum at upper pancreas, find trunk splenic artery, and block the trunk by splenic pedicle blocking clamp, so dissecting of hilus lienis vessels becomes easy. Divide goal location vessels and discontinuously loose hilus lienis block clip accompanied with laparoscopic ultrasound to assess the zone of ischemia to accurately excise lesions. Blocking the trunk of splenic artery when disconnecting spleen could lead to "auto transfusion" of blood in the spleen; meanwhile, a decrease in bleeding during disconnection of spleen or dissecting of hilus lienis was proved in our previous study [23]. For many patients with traumatic spleen rupture undergoing laparoscopic partial splenectomy, firstly we should aspirate blood around the spleen to expose the whole spleen; secondly we should assess the injury degree of spleen. We do not recommend patients with spleen pedicle injury and massive bleeding to undergo laparoscopic partial splenectomy. We suggest conducting selective splenic pedicle occlusion to patients with small vessel injury or less bleeding in spleen. Open retroperitoneum at upper pancreas, find trunk splenic artery, and block the trunk by splenic pedicle blocking clamp. Then conduct regional vessel and spleen dissection and blocking, and carry out auto transfusion of hematocoelia after excluding the liver, pancreas, and organ injury.

8.8.4 Time Limit of Splenic Artery Occlusion

The blood supply of spleen is mainly from splenic artery, greater curvature, and lower splenic omentum hemal arch. In the procedure of laparoscopic partial splenectomy, the inferior pole of spleen is supplied with blood by omentum hemal arch after blocking the flow of splenic artery and short gastric vessel. The anterior pole of spleen is supplied with blood by short gastric vessel after blocking the flow of omentum hemal arch vessel. So it will not result in ischemia of whole spleen. Teperman et al. reported that blocking for 2 h will not affect the spleen function [24]. In our center, the discontinuous occlusion is limited to 1 h [23], which lays the theoretical basis for conducting selective splenic pedicle occlusion.

8.8.5 Disconnection of Spleen and Dissociation of Ligament

The spreading of laparoscopic partial splenectomy benefits from the development of surgical instruments. Patients benefit from minimally invasive surgery with less injury, fast recovery, less morbidity, and reserving of organ function. The main methods to disconnect spleen include ultrasound scalpel, LigaSure, radiofrequency ablation, and Endo-GIA stapler. However, the key procedure to reduce bleeding in the operation is disconnecting spleen in the ischemia zone. Meanwhile the ischemia spleen should not be reserved too much; otherwise, complications such as stomachache, spleen necrosis, and infection may occur. We suggest dissecting spleen 0.5–1 cm to the ischemia line in the ischemia zone. For lesions located in the inferior pole of spleen, we should sufficiently dissociate the inferior pole of spleen, reserving the upper of spleen-stomach ligament, especially maintaining the completeness of short gastric vessel while reserving the splenophrenic ligaments. Pre-excise the anterior pole of spleen and keep the completeness of splenocolic ligament because it can preserve uninjured side blood supply and prevent spleen pedicle reversing after operation. If the uninjured side spleen is highly active with long spleen pedicle, fix the spleen can be conducted to prevent the postoperative spleen pedicle reversing. Fix the spleen pedicle and surrounding tissue on belly wall or omentum by 5-0 prolene. These complications rarely happen because the spleen adheres to surrounding tissue after surgery.

8.8.6 Disadvantages of Laparoscopic Partial Splenectomy

Laparoscopic partial splenectomy is a hard and high-risk operation. Operator needs a long study curve to successfully conduct this operation. Meanwhile surgical teams should have ability to handle intraoperative bleeding and other complications. Excessive reservation of ischemic tissue would lead to spleen necrosis, infection, abscess, stomachache, and fever. Currently the assessment of splenic function is expensive and complex, so laparoscopic partial splenectomy has not been widely conducted in many hospitals.

8.8.7 Future Prospects

Laparoscopic partial splenectomy needs proficient laparoscopic operation skills and tacit cooperation, so laparoscopic simulation training and instruction from experienced laparoscopic operator are important. Accurate preoperative assessment of the distribution of vessels, the volume of lesion and the rest volume of spleen, selective splenic pedicle occlusion, and identification of simple indicators for splenic function assessment are the future goals of laparoscopic partial splenectomy. Laparoscopic partial splenectomy represents contemporary idea of precision medicine to benefit patients much, including reservation of the organ function and less invasion. With the development of laparoscopic technique and renewed idea of surgery, laparoscopic partial splenectomy will have a better chance of advancement.

References

1. Breitenstein S, Scholz T, Schafer M, et al. Laparoscopic partial splenectomy. J Am Coll Surg. 2007;204(1):179–81.
2. Di Sabatino A, Carsetti R, Corazza G. Post-splenectomy and hyposplenic states. Lancet. 2011;378(9785):86–97.
3. Jais X, Ioos V, Jardim C, et al. Splenectomy and chronic thromboembolic pulmonary hypertension. Thorax. 2005;60(12):1031–4.
4. Hoeper M, Niedermeyer J, Hoffmeyer F, et al. Pulmonary hypertension after splenectomy? Ann Intern Med. 1999;130(6):506–9.
5. Hassn AM, Al-Fallouji MA, Ouf TI, et al. Portal vein thrombosis following splenectomy. Br J Surg. 2000;87(3):362–73.
6. Timens W, Leemans R. Splenic autotransplantation and the immune system. Adequate testing required for assessment of effect. Ann Surg. 1992;215(3):256–60.
7. Guan Y, Hu Y. Clinical application of partial splenic embolization. Sci World J. 2014;2014(3):1–9.
8. Morgenstem L, Shapiro SJ. Partial splenectomy for nonparasitic splenic cysts. Am J Surg. 1980;139(2):278–81.
9. [illegible] B, Sauerland S, Decker G, et al. Laparoscopic splenectomy: the clinical practice guidelines of the European Association for Endoscopic Surgery (EAES). Surg Endosc. 2008;22(4):821–48.
10. Coccolini F, Montori G, Catena F, et al. Splenic trauma: WSES classification and guidelines for adult and pediatric patients. World J Emerg Surg. 2017;12(1):1–40.
11. Ikeda M, Sekimoto M, Takiguchi S, et al. High incidence of thrombosis of the portal venous system after laparoscopic splenectomy: a prospective study with contrast-enhanced CT scan. Ann Surg. 2005;241(2):208–16.
12. van't Kiet M, Burger J, Van Muiswinkel J, et al. Diagnosis and treatment of portal vein thrombosis following splenectomy. Br J Surg. 2000;87(9):1229–33.
13. Liu DL, Xia S, Xu W, et al. Anatomy of vasculature of 850 spleen specimens and its application in partial splenectomy. Surgery. 1996;119(1):27–33.
14. Poulin EC, Schlachta CM, Mamazza J. Partial splenectomy, open and laparoscopic. Atlas of upper gastrointestinal and hepato-pancreato-biliary surgery. New York: Springer Press; 2016. p. 1047–52.
15. Kristinsson SY, Gridley G, Hoover RN, et al. Long-term risks after splenectomy among 8,149 cancer-free American veterans: a cohort study with up to 27 years follow-up. Haematologica. 2014;99(2):392–8.
16. Stoehr GA, Stauffer UG, Eber SW. Near-total splenectomy: a new technique for the management of hereditary spherocytosis. Ann Surg. 2005;241(1):40–7.
17. Lee SH, Lee JS, Yoon YC, et al. Role of laparoscopic partial splenectomy for tumorous lesions of the spleen. J Gastrointest Surg. 2015;19(6):1052–8.
18. Uranues S, Grossman D, Ludwig L, et al. Laparoscopic partial splenectomy. Surg Endosc. 2007;21(1):57–60.
19. Olthof DC, van der Vlies CH, Goslings JC. Evidence-based management and controversies in blunt splenic trauma. Curr Trauma Rep. 2017;3(1):32–7.
20. Brugere C, Arvieux C, Dubuisson V, et al. Early embolization in the non-operative management of blunt splenic injuries: a retrospective multicenter study. J Chir. 2008;145(2):126–32.
21. Moreno P, Von Allmen M, Haltmeier T, et al. Long-term follow-up after non-operative management of blunt splenic and liver injuries: a questionnaire-based survey. World J Surg. 2018;42(5):1358–63.
22. Li YB, Wang YC, Wang X, et al. Application of selective splenic pedicle occlusion in laparoscopic splenectomy. Chin J Gen Surg. 2017;32(2):122–5.
23. Balaphas A, Buchs NC, Meyer J, et al. Partial splenectomy in the era of minimally invasive surgery: the current laparoscopic and robotic experiences. Surg Endosc. 2015;29(12):3618–27.
24. Teperman SH, Whitehouse BS, Sammarlano RJ, et al. Bloodless splenic surgery: the safe warm-ischemic time. J Pediatr Surg. 1994;29(1):88–92.

Laparoscopic Splenectomy Combined Selective Pericardial Devascularization

9

Yongbin Li, Xin Wang, Haojun Wu, Jun Xu, Jiaying You, and Bing Peng

9.1 Background

Portal hypertension (PH), most often caused by cirrhosis, refers to a series of clinical syndromes characterized by the increased blood pressure of the portal vein system. It is often complicated by splenomegaly and varices. The bleeding of esophageal and gastric varices is the most important cause of death for patients with cirrhosis and portal hypertension, with the death rate of 30–50% [1]. Splenectomy plus pericardial devascularization is used to treat portal hypertension implicated with severe hypersplenism and esophagogastric bleeding varices, with the advantages of safe and effective haemostasis and low long-term recurrence rate [2]. After an in-depth study on the local anatomy of the cardiac region and the gastric coronary vein, Yang Zhen et al. advocated selective pericardial vascular devascularization which maintains the main stem of the coronary vein and the esophageal collateral vein and only removes the perforating vessels outside the serosa of the esophageal and cardiac region, so as to achieve complete devascularization and maintain spontaneous shunt [3].

In recent years, with the rapid development of laparoscopic technology and instruments, laparoscopic splenectomy combined selective peripheral cardiac devascularization (LSSPD) has become possible. Compared with the traditional open surgery, LSSPD, with the help of laparoscope, can provide a better visual field and more definite observation of the anatomical structure and facilitate more precise operation, so that laparoscopic surgery can disconnect the high esophageal branch and the ectopic esophageal branch thoroughly [4–7]. In this chapter, combined with the existing literatures, we are glad to share our team's experience in developing LSSPD to treat splenomegaly with hypersplenism and gastroesophageal variceal bleeding.

Y. Li · X. Wang · H. Wu · J. Xu · J. You · B. Peng (✉)
West China Hospital, Sichuan University, Chengdu, China

9.2 Indications and Contraindications

9.2.1 Indications

Splenectomy is applied to treat PH complicated with splenomegaly and hypersplenism, whose splenectomy criteria are according to those proposed by Watanabe's [8, 9]. The indications for laparoscopic splenectomy to treat portal hypertension with splenomegaly and hypersplenism are consistent with open ones. In consideration of the spleen size, perisplenic adhesion, and operators' experience, total laparoscopic or hand-assisted

B. Peng (ed.), *Laparoscopic Surgery of the Spleen*, https://doi.org/10.1007/978-981-16-1216-9_9

laparoscopic splenectomy can be chosen. The splenectomy criteria are listed below:

1. Platelets (PLT) <30 × 10^9/L and white blood cell (WBC) <3 × 10^9/L.
2. Platelets (PLT) <30 × 10^9/L or white blood cell (WBC) <3 × 10^9/L.
3. Bleeding from esophagogastric varices caused by various reasons, including rebleeding after repeated endoscopic treatment, with "red signs" revealed in gastroscopy and more likely to bleed recently [1].
4. Child-Pugh class A or B liver function.
5. Patients are able to tolerate general anesthesia and pneumoperitoneum for laparoscopic surgery.

9.2.2 Contraindications

Laparoscopic splenectomy is not recommended for patients whose hypersplenism is not serious enough to reach the abovementioned splenectomy criteria or who have extensive collateral circulation around the spleen with higher risk of splenectom [8, 10, 11]. The contraindications for the surgery are listed below:

1. Child-Pugh class C liver function.
2. Hepatic encephalopathy, severe coagulation dysfunction, severe jaundice, and refractory ascites.
3. Patients who are unable to tolerate general anesthesia and pneumoperitoneum because of severe cardiac, cerebral, pulmonary, or renal dysfunction.
4. Prophylactic devascularization should not be performed for mild to moderate varices without history of bleeding.
5. Extensive thrombosis of portal vein, superior mesenteric vein, and splenic vein.

9.3 Preoperative Assessment and Preparation

9.3.1 General Assessment

Routine tests on blood routine, coagulation function, hepatic and renal function, blood biochemistry, blood type, transfusion-transmitted diseases, and electrocardiogram should be performed. Fecal routine examination and occult blood examination indicate whether there is gastrointestinal bleeding. Upper endoscopy assists to estimate the degree of varicose vessels and the risk of bleeding. If necessary, further examinations such as echocardiography, pulmonary function test, dynamic electrocardiogram, and enteroscopy could be considered. To correct anemia and poor coagulation, transfuse red blood cell suspension and fresh frozen plasma combined with vitamin K intramuscular injection, respectively. And prescribe liver-protecting drugs to improve liver function, when necessary. Limit sodium intake lower 2 g daily and take oral diuretics. Nonselective β-blockers can be administered orally after ruling out contraindications such as sinus bradycardia, atrioventricular block, and bronchial asthma [12].

9.3.2 Imaging Assessment

1. Ultrasound of abdomen should be arranged in order to preliminarily judge the size of spleen and the amount of ascites and to rule out gallstones, space-occupying lesion in the liver and thrombosis of portal vein, superior mesenteric vein, and splenic vein.
2. Enhanced CT scan of upper abdomen can assess the size of the spleen, the degree of collateral circulation, and the inflammatory adhesions around the spleen further. Three-dimensional reconstruction of epigastric vessels can clearly indicate the varicose vessels and thrombus in the portal vein system so that detailed surgical strategies can be formed.

9.4 Surgical Procedures

9.4.1 Surgical Position and Surgeon Position

The patient is placed in a modified right lateral decubitus position, while head is higher than feet. The optimal angle is 30°–45° between the patient's back and the operating room table. Laparoscope is introduced into the abdominal cavity through 10 mm trocar in periumbilical region. Pneumoperitoneum is attained, using carbon dioxide gas to a pressure of 13 mmHg. A 12 mm trocar is placed inferior to the left costal margin in the midclavicular line as the main working port. A 5 mm trocar left and inferior to the xiphoid is for the surgeon's left-hand instrument. Another 5 mm trocar inferior to the costal margin in the left anterior axillary line is placed for the assistant's working port (Fig. 9.1). Port placement will need to be individualized to the patient's anatomy. For massive splenomegaly, the trocar placement is the same as that in Chap. 5.

9.4.2 Main Steps

9.4.2.1 Dissecting the Blood Vessels of Greater Gastric Curvature

After a thorough search of the abdominal cavity for the presence of splenic accessory, use an ultrasound knife or LigaSure electrotome to open gastrosplenic ligament so that the vascular arch of greater gastric curvature is exposed. If the gastrosplenic ligament is too thick, start with avascular area of gastrocolic ligament as an alternative. Next clamp and sever the vascular arch using Hem-o-lok. Then sever the varicose left gastroepiploic vein, the short gastric vein (Fig. 9.2), and left inferior phrenic vein (Fig. 9.3) along the greater gastric curvature from the bottom to the cardia. Dissect the splenodiaphragmatic ligament and upper part of splenorenal ligament simultaneously.

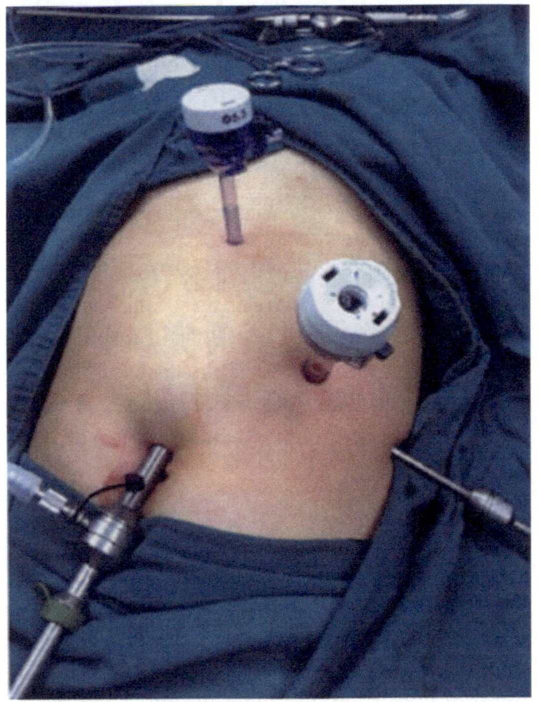

Fig. 9.1 Trocar placement

9.4.2.2 Amputating the Posterior Gastric Vessels

Grasp the posterior wall of the stomach, pull it to right to expose the varicose posterior gastric vein (Fig. 9.4), and amputate the vein using LigaSure

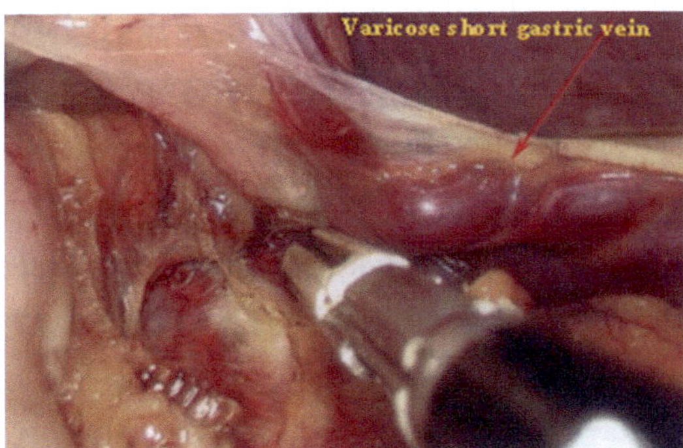

Fig. 9.2 Varicose short gastric vein

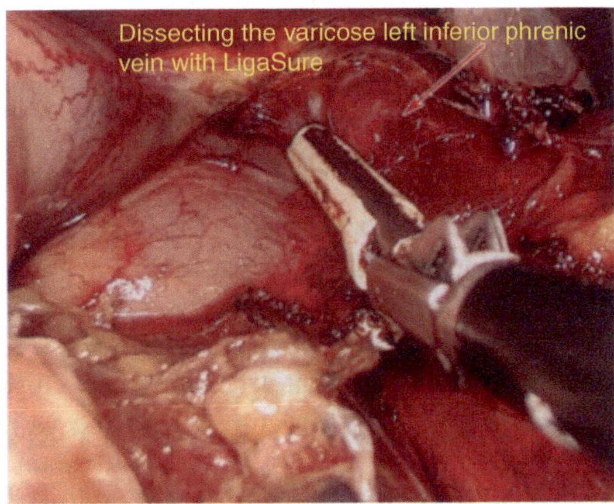

Fig. 9.3 Dissecting the varicose left inferior phrenic vein with LigaSure

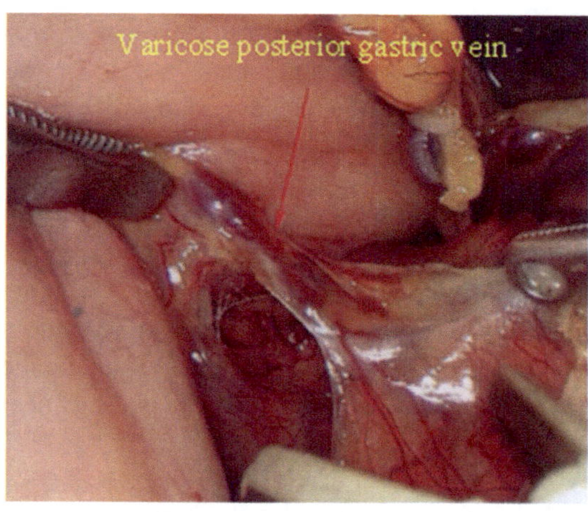

Fig. 9.4 Varicose posterior gastric vein

electrotome. Then open the posterior wall of the lesser omental bursa to expose the posterior gastric artery, sever the artery, and dissect upward to the posterior part of the cardia.

9.4.2.3 Dissociating the Inferior Pole of the Spleen

As the surgeon separates the splenocolic ligaments and the lower part of splenorenal ligament, traction and countertraction should be provided by the surgeon's nondominant hand and one hand of the assistant. Then cut the omentum tissue around the spleen to free splenic pedicle well.

9.4.2.4 Dissociating the Splenic Pedicle

The pedicle is transected using a linear vascular stapler. The work should be well visualized as the stapler is applied to avoid injury and sever completely. After transecting the splenic pedicle, the blood in the spleen can be used for autotransfusion.

9.4.2.5 Devascularizing the Perforator Veins of Gastric Lesser Curvature

While suspending the left lateral lobe of the liver (Fig. 9.5), penetrate the omentum close to the lesser gastric curvature where the varices are unmarked (Fig. 9.6) with an ultrasound knife. Then go through the hole with a urinary catheter to pull the stomach to left (Fig. 9.7).

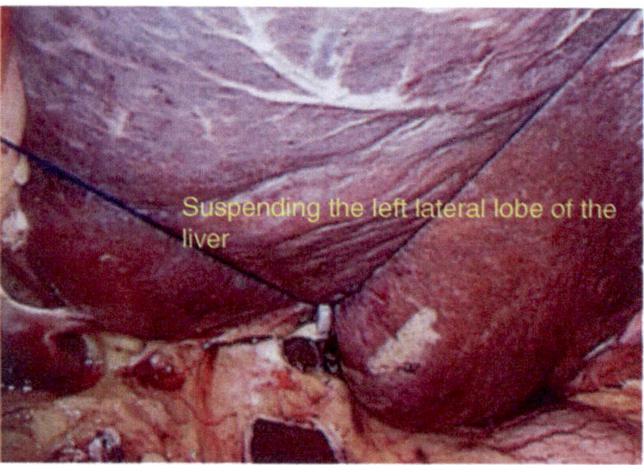

Fig. 9.5 Suspending the left lateral lobe of the liver

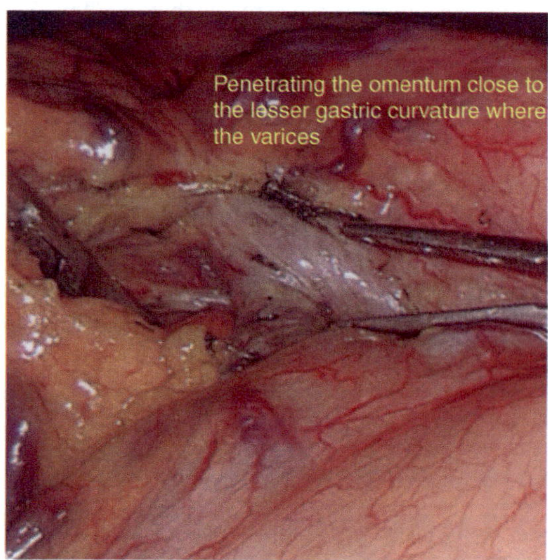

Fig. 9.6 Penetrating the omentum close to the lesser gastric curvature where the varices

Sever the gastric perforating branches of the gastric coronary vein (Fig. 9.8) along the lesser gastric curvature to the right crus of the diaphragm with LigaSure electrotome, whereas reserve the main trunk of the gastric coronary vein (Fig. 9.9).

9.4.2.6 Devascularizing the Perforator Veins of Esophagus

Open the anterior serosa of the subphrenic esophagus, and sever the esophagocardial varicose vein upward to the esophageal fissure of the diaphragm with LigaSure electrotome. Then devas-

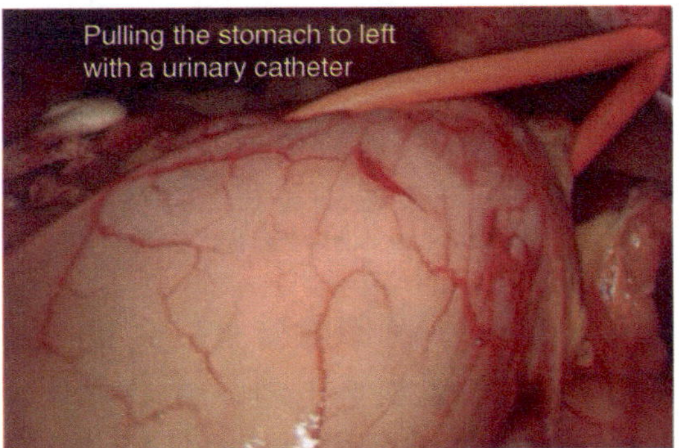

Fig. 9.7 Pulling the stomach to left with a urinary catheter

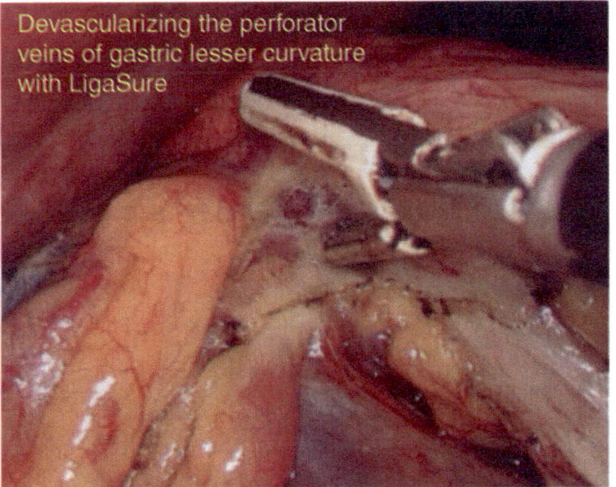

Fig. 9.8 Devascularizing the perforator veins of gastric lesser curvature with LigaSure

cularize the perforating vein of the esophagus by 5–10 cm close to the esophageal wall upward at the space between the crura of the diaphragm and the esophagus, including the high esophageal branch and the ectopic esophageal branch (Fig. 9.10), and reserve the integrity of the paraesophageal vein.

9.4.2.7 Taking the Specimen and Placing the Drainage Tube

Put the spleen specimen into a bag, and exteriorize the encased spleen through the periumbilical incision after fragmentation. Then take liver biopsy. After hemostasis, place a closed suction drain into the splenic fossa to complete the operation.

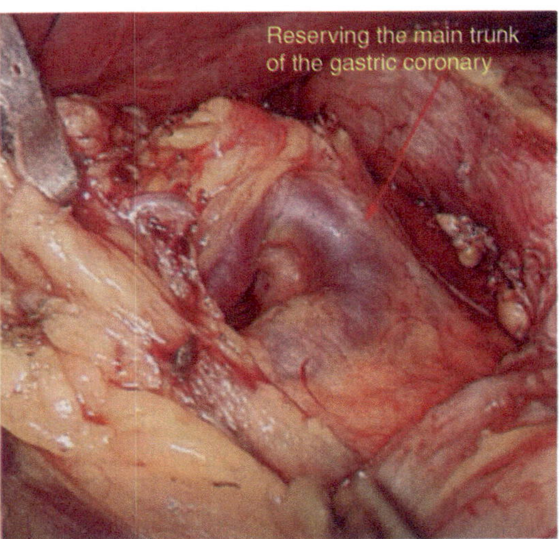

Fig. 9.9 Reserving the main trunk of the gastric coronary vein

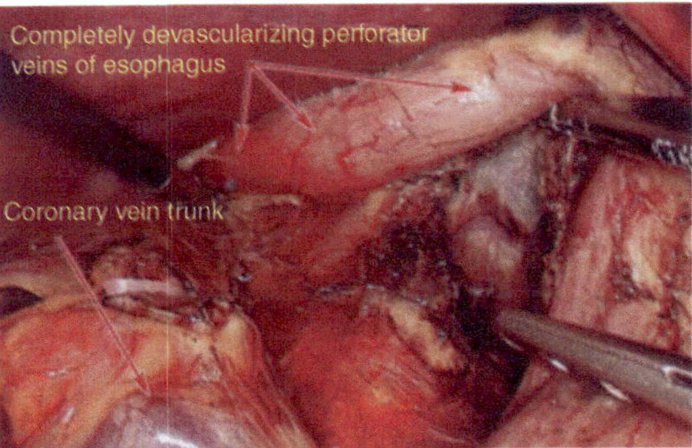

Fig. 9.10 Completely devascularizing the perforator veins of the esophagus

9.5 Key Surgical Techniques

9.5.1 Pericardial Devascularization

The development of electrosurgical devices is indispensable for laparoscopic pericardial devascularization. For example, LigaSure has better hemostatic effect than ultrasonic scalpel and can reduce the intraoperative use of Endo-GIA stapler and hemostatic clip, making the surgical vision clearer and more satisfactory. In addition, for the short gastric vessels which are more prone to bleeding, after the separation of the posterior area, the Hem-o-lok can be used for clipping at the spleen side if the short gastric vessels are short, and then LigaSure can be used for coagulation at the gastric wall side. Suture can also be used if the hemostasis effect is not as expected.

9.5.2 Blood Autotransfusion

Patients with portal hypertension are often complicated with anemia. However, there is more blood in the increscent spleen. Autotransfusion of blood in the resected spleen can not only correct the anemia but reduce a variety of complications caused by allogeneic blood transfusion. Besides, medical resources can be saved.

9.5.3 Hemostasis of Surgical Wound

Because of larger areas of surgical wound, higher portal hypertension, and poorer coagulation function, it is inefficient during operation using general electrocoagulation. Therefore, vascular suture can be used to stop bleeding completely.

9.6 Special Intraoperative Circumstances and Handling Skills

9.6.1 Bleeding

As a result of obvious portal hypertension complicated with varices, thrombocytopenia, and poor coagulation function, the patients with liver cirrhosis have a higher risk of bleeding than those without liver cirrhosis. It is difficult to control bleeding once hemorrhage occurs because of unclear operation area. Massive intraoperative bleeding is one of the main reasons for the conversion to laparotomy, with the conversion rate reported in the literature of 5.1–33.3% [6, 13]. The most serious condition is splenic pedicle bleeding, which will induce hemorrhagic shock rapidly; second, because of the remarkably swollen spleen and inflammatory adhesions around the short gastric vessels, perisplenic varicose vascular injury bleeding might occur commonly in short gastric vessels; finally, splenic injury and devascularization vascular bleeding are also dangerous.

9.6.1.1 Handling Skills for Splenic Pedicle Injury

The same as those of laparoscopic splenectomy in Chap. 5.

9.6.1.2 Handling Skills for Injury of Short Gastric Vessels

Due to the obvious short gastric varicose veins and high vascular pressure in liver cirrhosis, once bleeding occurs, the consequence is serious. So, manipulation should be gentle and careful during the operation. Our experience is opening the peritoneum of the posterior wall along the upper edge of the pancreas first, then pinching the main trunk of the splenic artery, and severing the posterior gastric vessels. After the separation of the posterior area of the short gastric vessels, cut off the short gastric vessels on the spleen and gastric wall sides using Hem-o-lok clipping and LigeSure, respectively. When the hemorrhage is difficult to control, it is necessary to convert to hand-assisted laparoscopic or open surgery.

9.6.1.3 Handling Skills for Bleeding due to Spleen Injury and Devascularization

For the handling skills for bleeding due to spleen injury, see Chap. 5 "Laparoscopic Splenectomy." During devascularization of pericardial vessels, LigaSure electrotome with the advantage of clearer operation vision and better hemostatic effect can reduce the use of cutting occluder and hemostatic clips during operation. For larger perforating vessels, suture hemostasis or Hem-o-lok clips can be used.

9.6.2 Adjacent Organ Injury

In addition to injury of diaphragm, stomach, colon, and pancreatic tail described in the previous chapters, the esophageal wall and parietal pleura may be damaged during devascularization of lower esophagus. When severing the perforating vein of the lower esophagus, going through the incorrect tissue space and the heat conduction of electrical surgical instruments may lead to the injury of esophageal sarcoplasmic layer. The instruments should walk through the gap between the left and right septal feet and esophagus and avoid clamping the esophageal wall. Once there is injury of esophagus, suture to repair. During transection of high esophageal branch and ectopic esophageal branch, LigaSure electrotome may incise the pleura near the esophagus resulting in pneumothorax. Once encountering pneumothorax, symptoms such as collapse of diaphragm, decrease in oxygen saturation, increase in airway pressure, and diminished breath sounds on the affected side can be found. In case of pleural injury, the surgeon should reduce the pneumoperitoneum pressure properly and suture the ruptured pleural fissure with vascular suture at the end of expiratory period with an anesthesiologist's ventilation.

9.7 Postoperative Management and Prevention and Treatment of Complications

9.7.1 Postoperative Management

The routine postoperative management is similar to that in Chap. 5.

It is necessary to prescribe oral diuretics and acid-suppressive drug and limit the intake of sodium and water after operation because of complications such as hypoalbuminemia, ascites, portal hypertensive gastric disease, and so on. Fresh frozen plasma infusion can be considered to the patients who have poor coagulation function and bleeding after operation. Patients with hypoalbuminemia can be intravenously infused with human serum albumin. Ultrasound examination of portal system should be performed routinely 5–7 days after surgery for patients who have a higher risk of portal vein thrombosis. Patients without the risk of bleeding are subcutaneously injected with low molecular weight heparin in order to prevent the portal vein thrombosis [14, 15].

9.7.2 Prevention and Treatment of Complications

9.7.2.1 Postoperative Hemorrhage

Early postoperative bleeding must be closely monitored, particularly in cirrhotic patients with poor coagulation function, portal hypertension, thrombocytopenia, and ascites. When the patients' hemodynamics is stable, mild hemorrhagic drainage might be caused by oozing from the surgical wound. It is necessary to apply hemostatic drugs, fresh frozen plasma, or red blood cell suspension timely according to fluctuations in hemoglobin levels. A large amount of bright red drainage combined with symptoms of hemorrhagic shock after operation is more likely to be macrovascular hemorrhage. It is necessary to have fluid infusion, transfusion, and emergency re-exploration at the same time.

9.7.2.2 Effusion of Splenic Fossa

Effusion of splenic fossa is a common complication in cirrhotic patients after splenectomy [13]. The management is the same as that in Chap. 5.

9.7.2.3 Pulmonary Complications

Pulmonary complications are often characterized by left pleural effusion and compressive atelectasis. The diagnosis and treatment are similar to those in Chap. 5.

9.7.2.4 Portal Vein Thrombosis

The incidence of portal vein thrombosis in cirrhotic patients is 20% [16] and can increase after splenectomy. The incidence after laparoscopic splenectomy is higher than that of traditional open one [17, 18], which is about 53.5–55% [14, 17]. Portal vein thrombosis can lead to upper gastrointestinal bleeding and liver failure. The diagnosis and treatment of portal vein thrombosis is similar to those in Chap. 5. When the effect of drug is poor, interventional therapy can be applied for fresh thrombus, while endovascular stent for old one [19, 20].

9.8 Hot Topics and Future Prospects

9.8.1 Theoretic Basis for Selective Pericardial Devascularization

Acute bleeding (incidence rate 50–80%) from ruptured esophagogastric varices is the serious cause of death in cirrhosis patients [21, 22]. Prevention and treatment of gastrointestinal bleeding from varices is the mainstay of the management of patients with portal hypertension. Although liver transplantation is the most effective treatment for patients with chronic decompensated cirrhosis, its widespread application is limited by organ shortage, high medical costs, and technical threshold. Splenectomy combined with devascularization of esophageal and gastric varices, with additional function for correcting the decrease of leukocytes and platelets caused by hypersplenism, can improve the prognosis of portal hypertension patients complicated with gastrointestinal hemorrhage [23, 24]. The traditional pericardial devascularization emphasizes blocking the blood flow of varices completely and thoroughly, whose procedure includes splenectomy, cutting short gastric vein, posterior gastric vein, left inferior phrenic vein, and main coronary vein of the stomach and even re-anastomosing the lower part of the esophagus after devascularization. However, this operation breaks the communication between portal vein system and gastric coronary vein, paraesophageal vein inferior pulmonary vein, azygos vein, and hemiazygos vein. As a result, the portal vein pressure is not decreased but increased, which leads to the recurrence of variceal bleeding and portal hypertensive gastropathy [25]. Therefore, the ideal operation should sever esophageal and gastric varices completely and reduce the impact on the blood circulation of portal vein system at the same time to avoid the recurrence of varices and gastrointestinal bleeding and minimize the risk of liver function deterioration.

Based on this, Yang Zhen proposed the selective devascularization around the esophagus and cardia, which disconnects the short gastric vein, the posterior gastric vein, the left inferior phrenic vein, gastric branch of gastric coronary vein, and the esophageal perforating veins of paraesophageal vein and keeps the integrity of trunks of gastric coronary vein and the paraesophageal vein to maintain the physiological portosystemic shunt. Compared with the traditional operation, the selective operation lowers the influence on the blood circulation of portal vein system and the risk of recurrence [3, 25]. Further, laparoscopic operation, with the following advantages of larger operation space formed by pneumoperitoneum and multiangle observation, is good at devascularization of high esophageal branch and ectopic esophageal branch which are prone to postoperative rebleeding. As a result of clearer field of vision and more accurate dissection, the occurrence of intraoperative injury and bleeding is reduced. In addition, laparoscopic operation is notable for minimal trauma, light pain, and quick recovery [6]. However, it has been reported that the incidence of portal vein thrombosis after laparoscopic splenectomy is higher than that after traditional open splenectomy [14, 17]. Therefore, it is important to monitor portal vein system in time after operation. Patients without anticoagulation taboo can be given low molecular weight heparin or warfarin. For patients with thromboembolism, thrombolysis or intravascular stent can be considered to improve the recanalization rate [15].

9.8.2 Advantages of LSSPD

The advantages of LSSPD includes (1) multiangle vision with the aid of high-definition laparoscope and the space established through pneumoperitoneum to provide a better surgical vision for LSSPD than the traditional open devascularization, especially for the devascularization of high and ectopic branches of lower esophagus susceptible to postoperative bleeding; (2) lower incidence of collateral injury and bleeding because of clearer vision and dissection; (3) less traction and stimulation on gastrointestinal tract and faster recovery of gastrointestinal function to allow for early liquid diet; and (4) small incision, light pain, early ambulation, faster recovery, and shorter hospital stay for saving medical resources.

9.8.3 Disadvantages of LSSPD

LSSPD is a highly risky and technically difficult operation, which requires a high professional level of the surgeons and surgical teams, especially when intraoperative hemorrhage occurs. Moreover, it is be reported in the literature that laparoscopic pneumoperitoneum pressure will increase the incidence of postoperative portal vein thrombosis and, in severe cases, will affect the postoperative liver function and even cause gastrointestinal bleeding. Therefore, a comprehensive assessment on the surgical experience of surgeons and operation conditions of hospitals shall be conducted before the LSSPD by putting the surgical safety in the first place.

9.8.4 Future Prospects

We should strengthen the simulation training on laparoscopic surgery and improve the capabilities of the surgical team for handling the abrupt hemorrhage during the operation. Higher access requirements should be put forward on the hospitals to conduct LSSPD. Meanwhile, to ensure the safety of laparoscopic splenectomy combined selective devascularization, we should strictly grasp the indications of operation preoperatively, especially for the patients with poor liver function and refractory ascites highly susceptible to preoperative or postoperative portal vein thrombosis. Due to the high incidence of perioperative complications and death, care should be taken for the operation, and looking for more reasonable and effective endoscopic or interventional treatment is the future development direction. Moreover, attention should be paid to timely identify the portal vein thrombosis and provide efficient treatment.

References

1. Public Health Industry Research Expert Group of the Health and Family Planning Commission. Expert consensus on technical specifications of treatment of portal hypertension with esophagogastric variceal bleeding (2013). Chinese J Digest Surg. 2014;13(6):401–4.
2. Yang LY. Current situation and prospect of surgical treatment on portal hypertension. Chinese J Digest Surg. 2015;14(1):10015–6.
3. Yang Z. Development and surgical techniques of selective pericardial devascularization. Chinese J Pract Surg. 2009;29(5):450–1.
4. Hong D, Cheng J, Wang Z, et al. Comparison of two laparoscopic splenectomy plus pericardial devascularization techniques for management of portal hypertension and hypersplenism. Surg Endosc. 2015;29(12):3819–26.
5. Kawanaka H, Akahoshi T, Kinjo N, et al. Laparoscopic splenectomy with technical standardization and selection criteria for standard or hand-assisted approach in 390 patients with liver cirrhosis and portal hypertension. J Am Coll Surg. 2015;221(2):354–66.
6. Zhe C, Jian-wei L, Jian C, et al. Laparoscopic versus open splenectomy and esophagogastric devascularization for bleeding varices or severe hypersplenism: a comparative study. J Gastrointest Surg. 2013;17(4):654–9.
7. Cai YQ, Zhou J, Chen XD, Wang YC, Wu Z, Peng B. Laparoscopic splenectomy is an effective and safe intervention for hypersplenism secondary to liver cirrhosis. Surg Endosc. 2011;25(12):3791–7.
8. Watanabe Y, Horiuchi A, Yoshida M, et al. Significance of laparoscopic splenectomy in patients with hypersplenism. World J Surg. 2007;31(3): 549–55.
9. Yang Z. Current situation and prospect of spleen surgery in the era of minimally invasive surgery. J Abdom Surg. 2015;28(6):377–81.
10. Jiang HC, Zhao XQ. Is splenectomy helpful or harmful for cirrhotic portal hypertension? Chin J Hepatobiliary Surg. 2006;12(9):581–3.
11. Xia SS. Careful selection of splenectomy should be emphasized for cirrhotic portal hypertension. Chin J Hepatobiliary Surg. 2006;12(9):583–4.
12. Garcia-Tsao G, Abraldes JG, Berxigotti A, et al. Portal hypertensive bleeding in cirrhosis: risk stratification, diagnosis, and management: 2016 practical guidance by the American Association for the study of liver diseases. Hepatology. 2017;65(1):310–35.
13. Li YB, Wang X, Wang YC, et al. Analysis of postoperative complications and risk factors in patients with portal hypertension treated by laparoscopic splenectomy. Chinese J Digest Surg. 2013;12(11):841–5.

14. de'Angelis N, Abdalla S, Lizzi V, et al. Incidence and predictors of portal and splenic vein thrombosis after pure laparoscopic splenectomy. Surgery. 2017;162(6):1219–30.
15. van't Riet M, Burger JW, van Muiswinkel JM, Kazemier G, Schipperus MR, Bonjer HJ. Diagnosis and treatment of portal vein thrombosis following splenectomy. Br J Surg. 2000;87(9):1229–33.
16. Lisman T, Violi F. Cirrhosis as a risk factor for venous thrombosis. Thromb Haemost. 2017;117(01):3–5.
17. Ikeda M, Sekimoto M, Takiguchi S, et al. High incidence of thrombosis of the portal venous system after laparoscopic splenectomy: a prospective study with contrast-enhanced CT scan. Ann Surg. 2005;241(2):208–16.
18. Kinjo N, Kawanaka H, Akahoshi T, et al. Risk factors for portal venous thrombosis after splenectomy in patients with cirrhosis and portal hypertension. Br J Surg. 2020;97(6):910–6.
19. Loffredo L, Pastori D, Farcomeni A, et al. Effects of anticoagulants in patients with cirrhosis and portal vein thrombosis: a systematic review and meta-analysis. Gastroenterology. 2017;153(2):480–7.
20. Valla DC, Condat B. Portal vein thrombosis in adults: pathophysiology, pathogenesis and management. J Hepatol. 2000;32(5):865–71.
21. Jensen DM. Endoscopic screening for varices in cirrhosis: findings, implications, and outcomes. Gastroenterology. 2002;122(6):1620.
22. Chinese Society of Portal Hypertension, Chinese Surgical Society, Chinese Medical Association. Consensus on diagnosis and treatment of cirrhotic portal hypertension with esophagogastric variceal bleeding (2015 edition). Chinese J Gen Surg. 2016;31(2):167–70.
23. Yamamoto N, Okano K, Oshima M, et al. Laparoscopic splenectomy for patients with liver cirrhosis: Improvement of liver function in patients with Child-Pugh class B. Surgery. 2015;158(6):1538–44.
24. Kawanaka H, Akahoshi T, Kinjo N, et al. Effect of laparoscopic splenectomy on portal haemodynamics in patients with liver cirrhosis and portal hypertension. Br J Surg. 2014;101(12):1585–93.
25. Hiroshi H, Yoshida H, Yasuhiro N, et al. New methods for the management of gastric varices. World J Gastroenterol. 2006;12(37):5926–31.

10 Laparoscopic Radical Antegrade Modular Pancreatosplenectomy

Pan Gao, Aihua Dong, and Bing Peng

10.1 Background

Distal pancreatic cancer has the characteristics of insidious onset, high malignancy, strong invasiveness, low R0 resection rate, and poor prognosis. The 5-year overall survival rate is lower than 5% [1]. Radical resection is still the only way to cure distal pancreatic cancer. R0 resection is the key factor affecting the long-term survival of patients [2–4]. Increasing the R0 resection rate of distal pancreatic cancer, delaying the time of recurrence, and reducing the local recurrence rate have always been hot topics and difficulties in pancreatic surgery research.

After the 1990s, with the continuous improvement of the concept of tumor treatment and surgical technology, the radical surgery of distal pancreatic cancer has been improved. After classic distal pancreatic cancer surgery, the positive rate of the retroperitoneal margin of the patient is high, which is an important reason of tumor metastasis and recurrence. In 2003, Strasberg et al. [5] first reported a new surgical method for distal pancreatic cancer—radical antegrade modular pancreatosplenectomy (RAMPS).

The original intention of RAMPS design is to increase the R0 resection rate of distal pancreatic cancer and reduce the positive rate of the posterior margin; at the same time, it can increase the number of lymph node dissections. Like pancreatic head cancer, distal pancreatic cancer is a highly malignant tumor with strong invasiveness, and it can easily break through the pancreatic capsule, invade the left adrenal gland, and even break through the renal fascia (also known as Gerota fascia) into the renal fat capsule. In traditional distal pancreatectomy, the separation level is between the posterior pancreas capsule and renal fascia, which can easily lead to tumor residual. RAMPS emphasizes a deeper level of resection, including renal fascia, prerenal fat sac, even the left adrenal gland, etc., so as to increase the rate of R0 resection and improve the patient's prognosis. Therefore, RAMPS attaches great importance to the radical resection of the posterior peritoneal margin. Based on the situation whether the tumor invades the posterior pancreatic capsule, the two types of RAMPS, inferior RAMPS and posterior RAMPS resection ranges, are used to improve the R0 resection rate of the posterior peritoneal margin and radical malignancy effect. If the tumor does not break through the posterior pancreatic fascia, anterior RAMPS is feasible, that is, the surgical removal plane is the surface of the left renal vein and the left adrenal gland for removing the posterior peritoneal tissue, and the distal pancreas, the spleen, and the left anterior renal fascia should be completely removed; if the tumor breaks through the dorsal pancreas of the pancreas, or even invades the left

P. Gao · A. Dong · B. Peng (✉)
West China Hospital, Sichuan University, Chengdu, China

B. Peng (ed.), *Laparoscopic Surgery of the Spleen*, https://doi.org/10.1007/978-981-16-1216-9_10

adrenal gland, posterior RAMPS is required, that is, the surgical removal plane is the surface of the left renal vein for removing the retroperitoneal tissue, and the left adrenal gland together with the distal pancreas, spleen, left kidney, and the anterior fascia should be completely removed.

Since 1999, the Strasberg team has published a series of important literatures about RAMPS [5–7]. Compared with the classic distal pancreatectomy and splenectomy, RAMPS has improved the R0 resection rate. Researches on RAMPS in Japan, South Korea, European countries, and other countries have been carried out successively, and significant clinical effects have been achieved [8–12]. With the rapid development of laparoscopic technology and further understanding of the posterior incisal margin of the pancreas and the drainage of peripancreatic lymph nodes, laparoscopic RAMPS has been widely used, and the feasibility, safety, and postoperative effect of laparoscopic RAMPS have been recognized [13, 14]. Undoubtedly, compared with traditional distal pancreatectomy and splenectomy and open RAMPS, laparoscopic RAMPS needs higher technical requirements and team cooperation requirements for the surgeon. Currently, only a few hospitals have reported laparoscopic or robot-assisted RAMPS [15–17], and most are reported as anterior RAMPS, which does not involve the total resection of the left adrenal gland [18, 19]. Posterior RAMPS has rarely been reported. The following sections will describe the experience of our team in laparoscopic RAMPS and show the laparoscopic RAMPS through the Treitz ligament approach by combining the existing literatures.

10.2 Indications and Contraindications

10.2.1 Indications

For the RAMPS surgical indications, RAMPS is suitable for patients with distal pancreatic cancer that is resectable or may be resected as diagnosed by pathological examination or clinical diagnosis (stage I–III according to American Cancer Association 8th edition TNM) [20] provided that there are no severe associated diseases that cannot tolerate surgery, distant metastasis, or locally vascular invasion that cannot undergo radical surgery. If the preoperative imaging examination or intraoperative judgment shows that the tumor does not invade the pancreatic capsule, anterior RAMPS should be chosen, and the modular resection plane is the surface of the left renal vein and left adrenal gland behind the Gerota fascia. If the tumor invades the pancreatic capsule, posterior RAMPS should be chosen, and the modular resection plane is along the surface of the left kidney behind the Gerota fascia and the left adrenal gland, with the left adrenal gland removed simultaneously.

Based on their own experience, Yonsei University in South Korea has proposed Yonsei criteria for the selection of minimally invasive RAMPS cases [19] (Yonsei criteria):

1. The tumor is confined in the pancreas.
2. A complete fascia layer can be seen between the distal pancreas and the left kidney and adrenal glands.
3. The distance between the tumor and the abdominal cavity is greater than 1 cm.

According to our center's own experience and technical characteristics, we think that both the anterior and posterior approaches of laparoscopic RAMPS are safe and feasible for patients with stage I–IIB pancreatic body and pancreatic tail cancer. For patients with stage IIIA tumors, laparoscopic pancreatic surgery can be performed in centers with rich experience.

10.2.2 Contraindications

1. Those with local blood vessels (abdominal cavity trunk and its branches, superior mesenteric artery, etc.) invaded and unable to undergo radical surgery
2. Those with distant metastasis
3. Those who cannot tolerate abdominal surgery due to various physical reasons

4. Those who cannot tolerate pneumoperitoneum due to cardiopulmonary dysfunction or other reasons

10.3 Preoperative Assessment and Preparation

Before surgery, patients should be sufficiently assessed for resectability by means of enhanced abdominal CT, MRI, etc., especially three-dimensional vascular reconstruction CT and CTA to sufficiently assess the relationship between the tumor and adjacent important blood vessels (abdominal trunk and its three branch arteries, superior mesenteric artery, the superior mesenteric vein, portal vein, inferior mesenteric vein, and splenic vein, the possibility of tumor invasion, and the possibility of vascular variability), so as to be clear whether vascular resection and reconstruction and RAMPS+Appleby surgery are necessary during the operation. PET-CT examination is provided when necessary to rule out the possibility of distant metastasis.

10.4 Surgical Procedures

Although laparoscopic RAMPS is more difficult than open RAMPS, laparoscopic surgery has greater advantages in certain aspects, such as small wounds and less pain. The magnifying effect of the laparoscope provides the surgeon with a clearer field of vision and a surgical angle that the laparotomy cannot provide, which makes the laparoscopic RAMPS more accurate and the resection more accurate. In traditional laparotomy, the surgeon obtains a surgical field from the ventral side to the dorsal side from top to bottom. In laparoscopic surgery, because of the anatomical position of the pancreas and the use of the laparoscopic 30° mirror, the entire surgical team can obtain dual surgical field of view from the foot side to the head side and from the ventral side to the dorsal side, so that the anatomical structure is revealed one by one and the intraoperative anatomy is more refined and precise.

Because of the special anatomical field of laparoscopic RAMPS, the laparoscopic RAMPS through the Treitz ligament approach can directly dissect and expose in turn the mesenteric veins, abdominal aorta, inferior vena cava, and left renal veins. The anatomical plane of the posterior Gerota fascia, the left adrenal gland, the left renal artery, the left renal vein, and the left kidney are excised together to complete the laparoscopic RAMPS. The specific surgical steps are as follows.

10.4.1 Surgical Position and Trocar Placement

Take the supine position, legs apart, head about 30° higher than feet (reverse Trendelenburg position), the left side slightly raised on with the left side higher than the right side. The main knife is located on the right side of the patient; one assistant is located on the left side of the patient and another assistant holding the laparoscope stands between the patient's legs.

The surgical method uses the classic "five-hole method" of pancreatic surgery (Fig. 10.1), and the five trocars surround the operation site in a semi-circular pattern. Take a 10 mm longitudinal incision under the navel as the observation

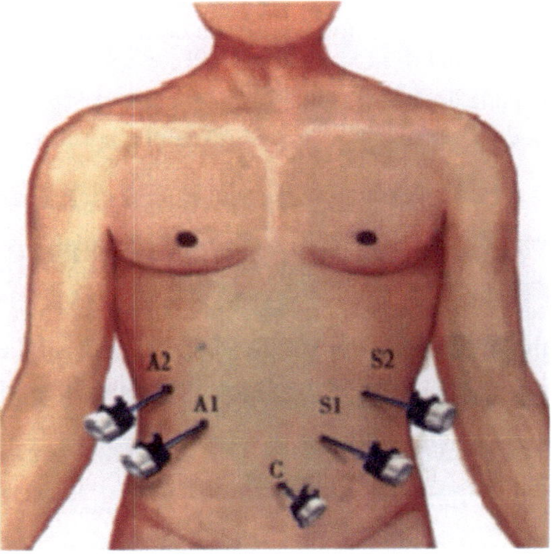

Fig. 10.1 Trocar placement

port (C), establish a carbon dioxide pneumoperitoneum, and control the pressure at about 13 mmHg. The remaining trocar holes are established under direct vision, and the remaining trocar holes are distributed as follows: S1 and A1 are symmetrically distributed at the lateral edge of the rectus abdominis muscle about 2 cm above the navel; S2 and A2 are symmetrically distributed under the costal margin of the anterior axillary line.

10.4.2 Exploration

Explore the abdominal cavity to rule out abdominal metastases.

10.4.3 Dissection of Upper and Lower Edges of the Pancreas

Use the ultrasonic scalpel to open the gastrointestinal ligament and the small omental sac on the side of the great curvature of the stomach. The urinary catheter is suspended on the stomach and pulled out under the xiphoid process, fully revealing the upper edge of the pancreas and confirming the location and size of the tumor. Open the upper edge of the pancreas with an ultrasonic scalpel, identify the running of the common hepatic artery, fully expose the common hepatic artery, and suspend the traction of the common hepatic artery. At the same time, clean the lymph nodes of group No. 8a, and reveal the portal vein at the upper edge of the pancreatic neck.

Use the ultrasonic scalpel to open the pancreas capsule along the lower edge of the pancreas, dissect layer by layer, separate and sever the left vessel of the gastric omentum, free and fully lower the splenic curvature of the colon, and reveal the lower edge of the pancreas. Expose the superior mesenteric vein at the lower edge at the neck of the pancreas.

10.4.4 Treitz Ligament Approach

Lift the transverse colon and mesentery to reveal the jejunum, free the jejunum up to the left side of the Treitz ligament along the proximal end of the jejunum, expose the inferior mesenteric vein, and disconnect it. Open the Treitz ligament and the surrounding mesentery, and after revealing the plane of the left renal vein, place a piece of gauze to confirm the anatomical plane and the position of the left renal vein (Fig. 10.2).

10.4.5 Disconnection of the Pancreas

Use the silk thread to lift the neck of the pancreas for pulling. Cut the closure device to disconnect the pancreas neck (Fig. 10.3), and squeeze the pancreas slowly for about 5 min before disconnecting the pancreas to reduce the risk of pancreatic fistula. After disconnection, check the pancreatic head for bleeding, and stop bleeding completely.

10.4.6 Spleen Movement, Venous Disconnection, and Local Lymph Node Dissection

After the pancreas is severed, the common hepatic artery is separated to the abdominal cavity, and

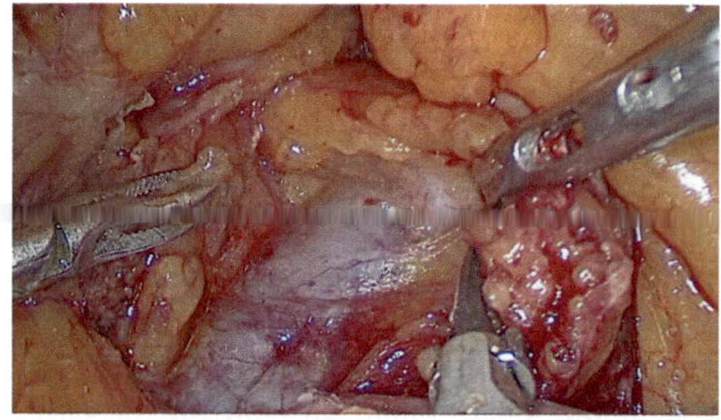

Fig. 10.2 Revealing the left renal vein through Treitz ligament

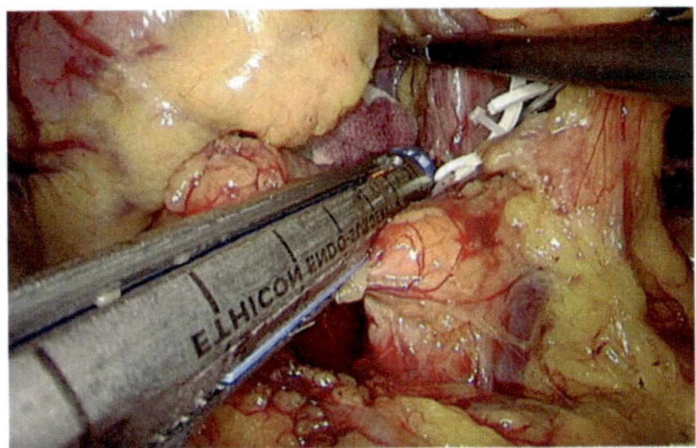

Fig. 10.3 Dissecting the splenic pedicle with an Endo-GIA

the coronary vein and the left gastric artery are severed at the root. The left common radius of the common hepatic artery and the abdominal cavity is exposed; the lymph nodes of groups No. 7, No. 8, and No. 9 are dissected; and then the root of the splenic artery is exposed. The splenic vein is cut off to expose the superior mesenteric artery, and the lymph nodes in front of the abdominal aorta between the root of the superior mesenteric artery and the abdominal cavity are cleaned.

10.4.7 Resection and Cleaning of Retroperitoneal Tissue

Dissect the left renal vein to the left to reveal the left adrenal artery, vein, left renal artery, and left renal surface. According to the depth of tumor invasion, decide whether to combine left adrenalectomy. Control the anatomical resection plane behind the Gerota fascia. If the tumor does not invade the posterior edge of the pancreas, proceed to the anterior approach RAMPS to remove the posterior peritoneal tissue close to the surface of the left renal vein and the left adrenal gland, and free the distal pancreas along the anterior retroperitoneal space of the left adrenal gland to the splenic hilum.

If the posterior edge of the pancreas is invaded, the posterior RAMPS is performed. After the left adrenal artery and vein are disconnected, the left adrenal gland is removed. Regardless of the anterior or posterior RAMPS, the left renal fascia and the prerenal fat sac need to be removed.

10.4.8 Spleen Dissociation

For the laparoscopic splenectomy, use the upper pole approach [21] to separate the spleen and stomach ligament and splenic septal ligament in turn and then the splenic colon ligament and spleen and kidney ligament, perform dissection to the splenic hilum, and complete the dissociation of the pancreatic body tail and spleen. Pancreatic body tail, spleen, peripheral lymph nodes, nerve fiber connective tissues around the blood vessels, and the posterior peritoneal tissue of the left Gerota fascia are completely excised, and the lymph node dissection of groups No. 10, No. 11, and No. 18 is completed (Figs. 10.4, 10.5, 10.6, and 10.7).

10.4.9 Taking the Specimen and Placing the Drainage Tube

After putting the specimen into the specimen bag, make a pneumoperitoneum incision under the umbilicus, and extend it 4 cm down to take out the specimen (Figs. 10.8 and 10.9). After closing

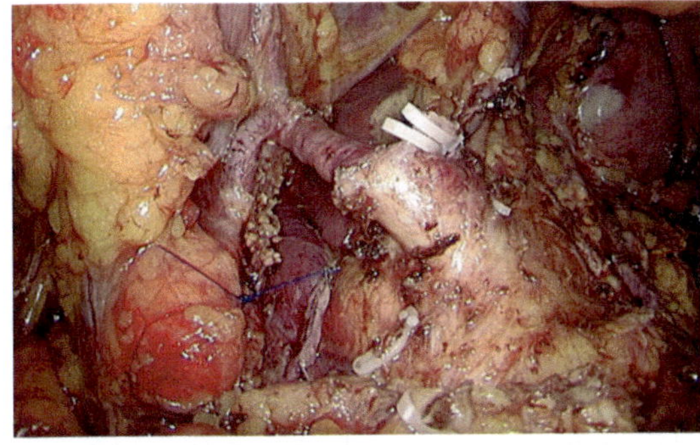

Fig. 10.4 After laparoscopic RAMPS dissection

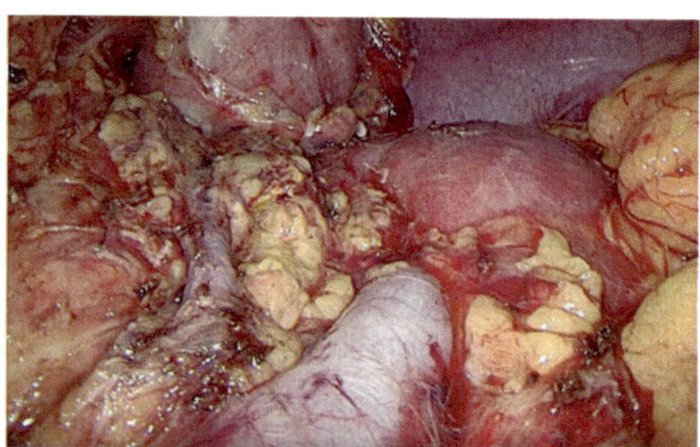

Fig. 10.5 Left renal vein and left kidney after laparoscopic RAMPS specimen excision

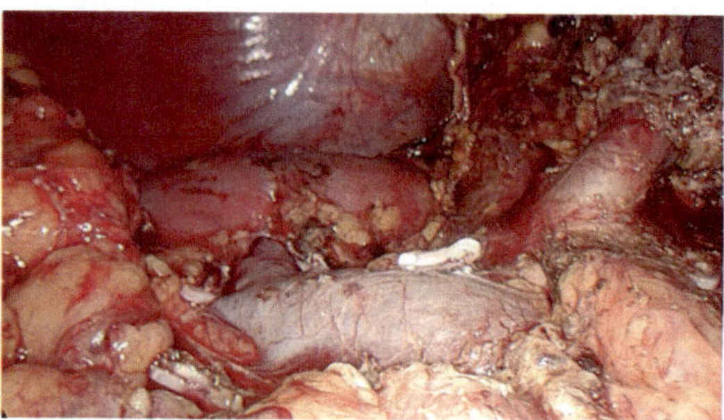

Fig. 10.6 Left renal vein and left kidney after laparoscopic RAMPS

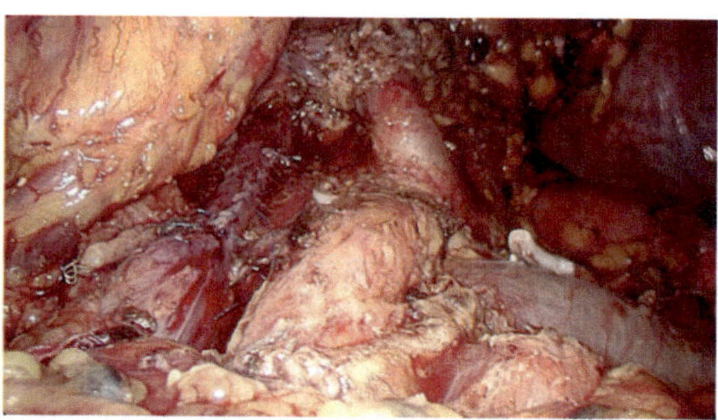

Fig. 10.7 After portal vein-superior mesenteric vein wedge resection and laparoscopic RAMPS dissection

the incision, build pneumoperitoneum, and completely stop the wound bleeding. After confirming that there is no significant active bleeding, place a drainage tube at the pancreatic stump and splenic fossa, and then lead it out through the trocar holes on the left and right sides (Fig. 10.10).

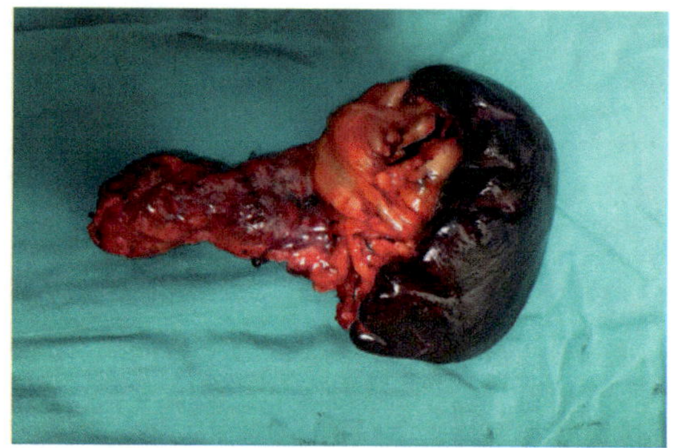

Fig. 10.8 Specimen after the surgery

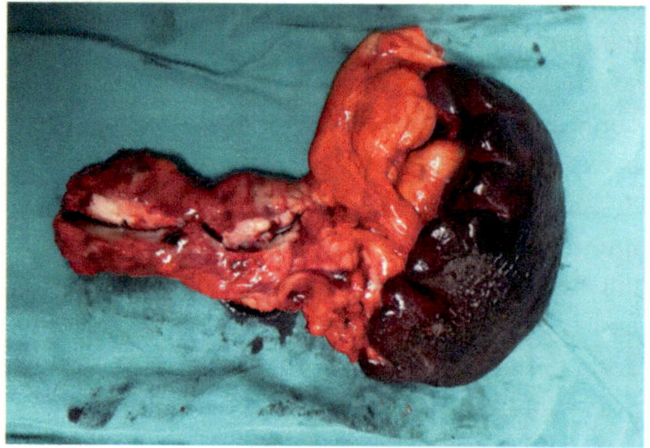

Fig. 10.9 Specimen after the surgery

10.5 Key Surgical Techniques

10.5.1 Anatomical Position and Resection Plane

In the traditional laparotomy for RAMPS, the feasible enlarged Kocher incision reveals the inferior vena cava, left renal vein, abdominal aorta, and superior mesenteric artery from right to left. When the RAMPS is performed under laparoscope, due to the change in the operation space, on the left side of the Treitz ligament, the inferior mesenteric vein can be exposed and severed. Then look for the left renal vein layer by layer, and expose the left renal vein. After confirming the location of the left renal vein, the anatomical layer (left renal vein and surface of the

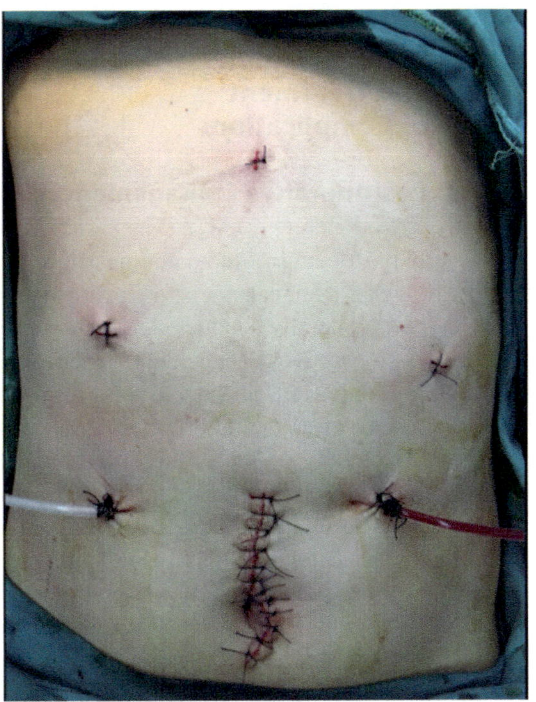

Fig. 10.10 Incision after the surgery

left kidney) and the direction of resection (from the root of the left renal vein to the left) can be determined. Because this procedure requires cleaning of the superior mesenteric artery and lymph nodes around the abdominal cavity, when the anatomy of the superior mesenteric artery is unchanged, the surgeon can search for the superior mesenteric artery above the left renal vein to facilitate identifying anatomical location and complete resection of the later specimen.

10.5.2 Protection of Renal Veins and Blood Vessels Around Renal Arteries

When operating along the surface of the left renal vein from right to left, the lumbar ascending vein at the lower edge of the left renal vein and the left testicular (ovarian) vein should be protected. The renal artery runs above and behind the renal vein and is divided into the front and back branches into the kidney at the renal hilum. Care should be taken to protect the renal arteries from damage, so as to avoid renal ischemic necrosis.

10.5.3 Treatment of Inferior Mesenteric Vein

The inferior mesenteric vein can merge into the splenic vein or superior mesenteric vein. In the case where the inferior mesenteric vein merges into the splenic vein, it can be disconnected at the lower edge of the pancreas at one time. If the inferior mesenteric vein merges into the superior mesenteric vein, the inferior mesenteric vein may run in front of the superior mesenteric artery. When handling the superior mesenteric artery during the operation, it is necessary to pay attention to the distribution of the inferior mesenteric vein and break off the inferior mesenteric vein at the junction of the superior and inferior mesenteric veins.

10.6 Special Intraoperative Circumstances and Handling Skills

10.6.1 Bleeding

When the key arteries and veins are released during the operation, the blood vessels can be suspended with a vascular sling to facilitate intraoperative traction and better reveal the anatomical structure. During intraoperative bleeding, blind clamping and ligation should be absolutely avoided. After fully revealing the surgical field of vision and the location of the bleeding, the most appropriate treatment method should be selected according to the situation. For active hemorrhage, precise ligation is the most accurate way to stop bleeding. If necessary, a blood vessel can be blocked to facilitate the exposure of the surgical field of vision and find the location of the bleeding. In case of bleeding at multiple spots, it is recommended to use gauze to compress them first, clear the surgical field of vision, then look for the locations of the bleeding, and deal with it one by one. In the case of bleeding that is difficult to handle under laparoscopy, it is recommended to transfer the laparotomy for hemostasis treatment in time to avoid further aggravation of the bleeding and ensure the safety of the patient.

10.6.2 Intraoperative Management of Pancreatic Stump

It is recommended to use a linear cutting device to cut off the neck of the pancreas and squeeze the pancreas slowly for 10–15 min before cutting off the pancreas. If the broken end of the main pancreatic duct is accurately found after severing, the broken end if seen can be sutured again. Prolene thread is recommended to be sutured routinely to reduce bleeding on the wound surface.

10.6.3 Anatomical Position and Resection Plane

During operation, the inferior mesenteric vein is exposed on the left side of the Treitz ligament, and it is severed. Then look for the left renal vein layer by layer, and expose the left renal vein. After confirming the location of the left renal vein, the anatomical layer (left renal vein and surface of the left kidney) and the direction of resection (from the root of the left renal vein to the left) can be determined. Because this procedure requires cleaning of the superior mesenteric artery and lymph nodes around the abdominal cavity, the superior mesenteric artery is generally located above the left renal vein when there is no variation in the superior mesenteric artery anatomy.

10.7 Postoperative Management and Prevention and Treatment of Complications

10.7.1 Postoperative Management

1. General postoperative treatment measures

   The general management of laparoscopic RAMPS is generally conducted in accordance with “Postoperative Management” in Chap. 5.
2. Routine monitoring on the 1st, 2nd, 3rd, 5th, and 7th day after operation should be conducted, including blood routine, biochemical complete set, blood coagulation function, procalcitonin, serum amylase, and lipase, and simultaneous detection of drainage fluid amylase and lipase to determine the presence of pancreatic fistula and its severity. On the 5th day after operation, the chest and abdomen CT and abdominal color Doppler ultrasound should be reviewed, and the patients undergoing vascular revascularization should be reexamined with CTA and portal vein Doppler ultrasound to understand the smooth blood flow of the portal vein system.
3. Prophylactic antibiotics can help reduce the infection-related mortality of surgery. Therefore, for patients undergoing pancreatic surgery, prophylactic antibiotics are recommended. In the absence of infection, antibiotics should be stopped within 72 h after surgery. In case of postoperative infection, antibiotics should be used according to the common source of infection at the site of infection and related culture results.
4. Preventive use of somatostatin and its analogs

   It is still controversial, and there is no unified conclusion that somatostatin can reduce the incidence of postoperative pancreatic fistula. The Cochrane systematic review updated in 2013 pointed out that although somatostatin analogs did not reduce perioperative mortality, they could significantly reduce perioperative complications, so it is recommended that somatostatin analogs be routinely used in the postoperative management of pancreatic surgery [22].

10.7.2 Prevention and Treatment of Postoperative Complications

10.7.2.1 Pancreatic Fistula

Pancreatic fistula is a common complication after distal pancreatectomy. Compared with laparoscopic splenectomy, the incidence of pancreatic fistula is higher and more harmful in distal pancreatectomy. It may cause serious complications such as bleeding, abdominal infection, multiple-organ failure, and death. After the occurrence of pancreatic fistula, maintaining good drainage is the first priority, and somatostatin analogues should be used for treatment. For patients with pancreatic fistula that causes abdominal infection, symptomatic treatment of antibiotics should be used in time, and the anti-infection program should be replaced in time according to the results of the culture of drainage fluid. Patients with severe sepsis and other organ failures should be treated by multidisciplinary treatment in a timely manner and surgical treatment if necessary.

10.7.2.2 Hemorrhage

The early bleeding in the abdominal cavity usually occurs within 24 h after the operation. Most of them are caused by incomplete hemostasis during the operation, and the operation should be stopped as soon as possible. Late bleeding usually occurs 10 days after surgery, mostly due to pancreatic fistula erosion of vascular end or pseudoaneurysm formation. Interventional methods should be used to identify the bleeding site, and embolization or stenting should be used to stop bleeding. If the intervention is invalid, surgical exploration should be done to stop bleeding.

10.7.2.3 Abdominal Infections

After pancreatic surgery, abdominal infections are often related to pancreatic fistulas. For patients suspected of abdominal infections, abdominal color Doppler ultrasound or abdominal CT examination should be performed in time to identify the infection site and assess whether puncture and drainage can be performed. For patients unable to undergo puncture and drainage, timely surgical drainage is necessary. Patients with pancreatic fistulas that cause abdominal infections should be treated symptomatically with antibiotics in a timely manner, and the anti-infection program should be replaced in time according to the results of the drainage fluid culture.

10.7.2.4 Postoperative Platelet Increase

Platelet increase within a few days after splenectomy and to the peak within 2 weeks can cause thrombosis in the brain, lungs, limbs, and mesentery. In case of postoperative platelet count $>400 \times 10^9$/L, when there is no obvious tendency of active bleeding, it is recommended to give antiplatelet aggregation drugs in a timely manner for symptomatic treatment, such as aspirin. After discharge from the hospital, regular monitoring of changes in platelet count is required to facilitate timely adjustment of the treatment plan.

10.7.2.5 Endocrine and Exocrine Insufficiency of Pancreatic Body and Tail After Surgery

The occurrence of endocrine and exocrine insufficiency of pancreatic body and tail after surgery varies from person to person, and patients with endocrine and exocrine insufficiency after surgery should be treated accordingly. For patients with high blood sugar after early recovery of diet, it is recommended to cooperate with endocrinologists to develop corresponding individualized hypoglycemic programs. For patients with pancreatic exocrine insufficiency, it is recommended to use exogenous digestive enzymes for pancreatin replacement therapy. The initial dose is usually 40,000–50,000 U/day. Thereafter, the dose should be adjusted according to the condition.

10.8 Hot Topics and Future Prospects

10.8.1 Sufficient Preoperative Assessment

There is currently no means to accurately assess whether pancreatic tumors invade blood vessels and the extent of invasion. At present, the most widely used assessment methods are three-dimensional reconstruction CT scan of the abdominal abdomen and enhanced MRI of the upper abdomen. Through the three-dimensional enhanced reconstruction CT, it is possible to determine whether the main blood vessels are mutated and invaded by tumor. Before the operation, our center will routinely perform enhanced CT scanning of three-dimensional reconstruction of blood vessels to understand the conditions of blood vessels. Common vascular variations include the origin of the right hepatic artery from the superior mesenteric artery and the absence of the common hepatic artery. Sufficient preoperative assessment can direct the operator to determine whether it is necessary to perform vascular resection and reconstruction and the possibility of RAMPS+Appleby surgery.

10.8.2 Safety of Laparoscopic RAMPS

Due to the difficulty of pancreatic surgery, the safety of laparoscopic RAMPS is one of the key concerns of pancreatic surgeons. RAMPS itself is more difficult than traditional surgical methods and requires more retroperitoneal dissection, vascular denudation, and lymph node dissection. Lee SH et al. from Yonsei University in Korea found that 12 selected pancreatic body and tail cancer patients received R0 resection after receiving minimally invasive RAMPS; compared with open surgery, the number of lymph nodes removed in the minimally invasive surgery group [(10.5 ± 7.1) vs. (13.8 ± 11.1), $P = 0.313$], postoperative complication rate (25% vs. 37.2%, $P = 0.412$), and median survival time (60 months vs. 61 months, $P = 0.616$, tendency score matching analysis results) had no difference, the surgery did not significantly increase the incidence of complications, and minimally invasive surgery helped shorten the length of hospital stay [(12.3 ± 6.8) day vs. (22.4 ± 21.6) day, $P = 0.002$] [19].

10.8.3 The Key to Improve R0 Resection Rate

R0 resection is an independent factor affecting the prognosis of patients with pancreatic body and tail cancer surgery [10]. Classical pancreatic body tail + splenectomy is the standard surgical method for the treatment of pancreatic body tail cancer [14]. However, due to pancreatic cancer anatomy and biological behavior characteristics, the R1 resection rate after radical pancreatic cancer surgery is as high as 76%, and the 5-year survival rate of patients after surgery is only 10%. Many patients have local recurrence early after surgery [14, 23]. This is related to the high positive rate (36–90%) of peritoneal resection margin [5, 24–26].

The original intention of RAMPS is designed as follows:

1. Improve the R0 resection rate of pancreatic body and tail cancer and reduce the positive rate of posterior margin.
2. Increase the number of lymph nodes removed. The purpose is to replace the classic pancreatic body tail + splenectomy and obtain a higher R0 resection rate.

The important purpose of RAMPS is to improve R0 resection rate. Therefore, it is particularly important to check the state of the cutting edge, especially the back cutting edge. Strasberg et al. [6] suggested that the posterior margin should be stained with ink and then checked to improve accuracy. In addition, a rapid pathological examination is recommended for the resection margin of the pancreas. For tumors that break through the pancreatic capsule without excluding nerve invaders, the SMA and the plexus at the abdominal cavity should be marked and examined separately. If the plexus at the SMA and the plexus in the abdominal cavity are not removed, a rapid pathological examination should be performed after biopsy.

10.8.4 Current Problems of RAMPS

According to current clinical research, RAMPS is also controversial and open to discussion [27–29]. At present, case-control studies on RAMPS and traditional surgery report that from the current research results, RAMPS does obtain a higher R0 resection rate (77–100%), but the recurrence rate is still high, and the long-term efficacy is still uncertain [9, 11, 14, 19, 30]. After RAMPS, pancreatic body and tail cancer still has a higher recurrence rate, of which systemic recurrence is more common than local recurrence. In theory, RAMPS may reduce the rate of local recurrence, but is not effective for systemic recurrence. However, according to the current data analysis, it is not easy to determine whether the local recurrence site is in the residual pancreas, tumor bed, or regional lymph nodes, which is one of the reasons why it is difficult to judge the actual effect of RAMPS.

10.8.5 Future Prospects

The progress in surgical treatment of pancreatic body and tail cancer is limited. The current research results show that RAMPS helps improve the R0 resection rate of pancreatic body and tail cancer, but the effect on tumor recurrence and long-term survival of patients is still uncertain. The long-term efficacy of RAMPS after minimally invasive techniques also needs further study. Therefore, a high-quality prospective, multi-center, randomized, and controlled study on laparoscopic surgery and traditional open surgery is the research direction in the future.

For the management of the perioperative period, whether preoperative treatment is meaningful for RAMPS, especially after the tumor breaks through the pancreatic fascia and the adrenal gland, remains to be discussed. In summary, these issues will be addressed in the high-quality clinical research in the future.

References

1. Hidalgo M. Pancreatic cancer. N Engl J Med. 2010;362(17):1605–17.
2. Marzano E, Piardi T, Soler L, et al. Augmented reality-guided artery-first pancreaticoduodenectomy. J Gastrointest Surg. 2013;17(11):1980–3.
3. Yamamoto T, Yagi S, Kinoshita H, et al. Long-term survival after resection of pancreatic cancer: a single-center retrospective analysis. World J Gastroenterol. 2015;21(1):262–8.
4. Hartwig W, Hackert T, Hinz U, et al. Pancreatic cancer surgery in the new millennium: better prediction of outcome. Ann Surg. 2011;254(2):311–9.
5. Strasberg SM, Drebin JA, Linehan D. Radical antegrade modular pancreatosplenectomy. Surgery. 2003;133(5):521–7.
6. Strasberg SM, Linehan DC, Hawkins WG. Radical antegrade modular pancreatosplenectomy procedure for adenocarcinoma of the body and tail of the pancreas: ability to obtain negative tangential margins. J Am Coll Surg. 2007;204(2):244–9.
7. Mitchem JB, Hamilton N, Gao F, et al. Long-term results of resection of adenocarcinoma of the body and tail of the pancreas using radical antegrade modular pancreatosplenectomy procedure. J Am Coll Surg. 2012;214(1):46–52.
8. Chang YR, Han SS, Park SJ, et al. Surgical outcome of pancreatic cancer using radical antegrade modular pancreatosplenectomy procedure. World J Gastroenterol. 2012;18(39):5595–600.
9. Kitagawa H, Tajima H, Nakagawara H, et al. A modification of radical antegrade modular pancreatosplenectomy for adenocarcinoma of the left pancreas: significance of en bloc resection including the anterior renal fascia. World J Surg. 2014;38(9):2448–54.
10. Rosso E, Langella S, Addeo P, et al. A safe technique for radical antegrade modular pancreatosplenectomy

with venous resection for pancreatic cancer. J Am Coll Surg. 2013;217(5):35–9.
11. Kang CM, Kim DH, Lee WJ. Ten years of experience with resection of left-sided pancreatic ductal adenocarcinoma: evolution and initial experience to a laparoscopic approach. Surg Endosc. 2010;24(7):1533–41.
12. Yamamoto J, Saiura A, Koga R, et al. Improved survival of left-sided pancreas cancer after surgery. Jpn J Clin Oncol. 2010;40(6):530–6.
13. Choi SH, Kang CM, Lee WJ, et al. Multimedia article. Laparoscopic modified anterior RAMPS in well-selected left-sided pancreatic cancer: technical feasibility and interim results. Surg Endosc. 2011;25(7):2360–1.
14. Kang CM, Lee SH, Lee WJ. Minimally invasive radical pancreatectomy for left-sided pancreatic cancer: current status and future perspectives. World J Gastroenterol. 2014;20(9):2343–51.
15. Abu Hilal M, Richardson JR, de Rooij T, et al. Laparoscopic radical 'no-touch' left pancreatosplenectomy for pancreatic ductal adenocarcinoma: technique and results. Surg Endosc. 2016;30(9):3830–8.
16. Kim EY, Hong TH. Initial experience with laparoscopic radical antegrade modular pancreatosplenectomy for left-sided pancreatic cancer in a single institution: technical aspects and oncological outcomes. BMC Surg. 2017;17(1):2–8.
17. Ome Y, Hashida K, Yokota M, et al. Laparoscopic radical antegrade modular pancreatosplenectomy for left-sided pancreatic cancer using the ligament of Treitz approach. Surg Endosc. 2017;31(11):4836–7.
18. Sunagawa H, Harumatsu T, Kinjo S, et al. Ligament of Treitz approach in laparoscopic modified radical antegrade modular pancreatosplenectomy: report of three cases. Asian J Endosc Surg. 2014;7(2):172–4.
19. Lee SH, Kang CM, Hwang HK, et al. Minimally invasive RAMPS in well-selected left-sided pancreatic cancer within Yonsei criteria: long-term (>median 3 years) oncologic outcomes. Surg Endosc. 2014;28(10):2848–55.
20. Kamarajah SK, Burns WR, Frankel TL, et al. Nathan H. Validation of the American Joint Commission on Cancer (AJCC) 8th Edition Staging System for Patients with Pancreatic Adenocarcinoma: a Surveillance, Epidemiology and End Results (SEER) analysis. Ann Surg Oncol. 2017;24(7):2023–30.
21. Cai YQ, Zhou J, Chen XD, et al. Laparoscopic splenectomy is an effective and safe intervention for hypersplenism secondary to liver cirrhosis. Surg Endosc. 2011;25(12):3791–7.
22. Gurusamy KS, Koti R, Fusai G, et al. Somatostatin analogues for pancreatic surgery. Cochrane Database Syst Rev. 2013;4:CD008370.
23. Esposito I, Kleeff J, Bergmann F, et al. Most pancreatic cancer resections are R1 resections. Ann Surg Oncol. 2008;15(6):1651–60.
24. Strasberg SM, Fields R. Left-sided pancreatic cancer: distal pancreatectomy and its variants: radical antegrade modular pancreatosplenectomy and distal pancreatectomy with celiac axis resection. Cancer J. 2012;18(6):562–70.
25. Westgaard A, Tafjord S, Farstad IN, et al. Resectable adenocarcinomas in the pancreatic head: the retroperitoneal resection margin is an independent prognostic factor. BMC Cancer. 2008;8(1):1–10.
26. Wu WG, Wu XS, Li ML, et al. Concept and strategy of antegrade pancreatectomy combined with splenectomy in radical resection of pancreas body and tail cancer. Chin J Pract Surg. 2015;35(3):296–8.
27. Iwagami Y, Eguchi H, Wada H, et al. Implications of peritoneal lavage cytology in resectable left-sided pancreatic cancer. Surg Today. 2015;45(4):444–50.
28. Hirabayashi K, Imoto A, Yamada M, et al. Positive intraoperative peritoneal lavage cytology is a negative prognostic factor in pancreatic ductal adenocarcinoma: a retrospective single-center study. Front Oncol. 2015;182(5):1–5.
29. Paiella S, Sandini M, Gianotti L, et al. The prognostic impact of para-aortic lymph node metastasis in pancreatic cancer: a systematic review and meta-analysis. Eur J Surg Oncol. 2016;42(5):616–24.
30. Kawabata Y, Hayashi H, Takai K, et al. Superior Mesenteric Artery-First Approach in Radical Antegrade Modular Pancreatosplenectomy for Borderline Resectable Pancreatic Cancer: A Technique to Obtain Negative Tangential Margins. J Am Coll Surg. 2015;220(5):49–54.

Correction to: Overview and Prospects of Laparoscopic Splenectomy

Xiaodong Chen, Shi Qiu, and Bing Peng

Correction to:
B. Peng (ed.), Laparoscopic Surgery of the Spleen,
https://doi.org/10.1007/978-981-16-1216-9_1

The affiliation of the author Xiaodong Chen was incorrect and has been revised to: Sichuan Cancer Hospital, School of Medicine, University of Electronic Science and Technology of China, Chengdu, China.

The updated online version of this chapter can be found at https://doi.org/10.1007/978-981-16-1216-9_1

B. Peng (ed.), *Laparoscopic Surgery of the Spleen*, https://doi.org/10.1007/978-981-16-1216-9_11

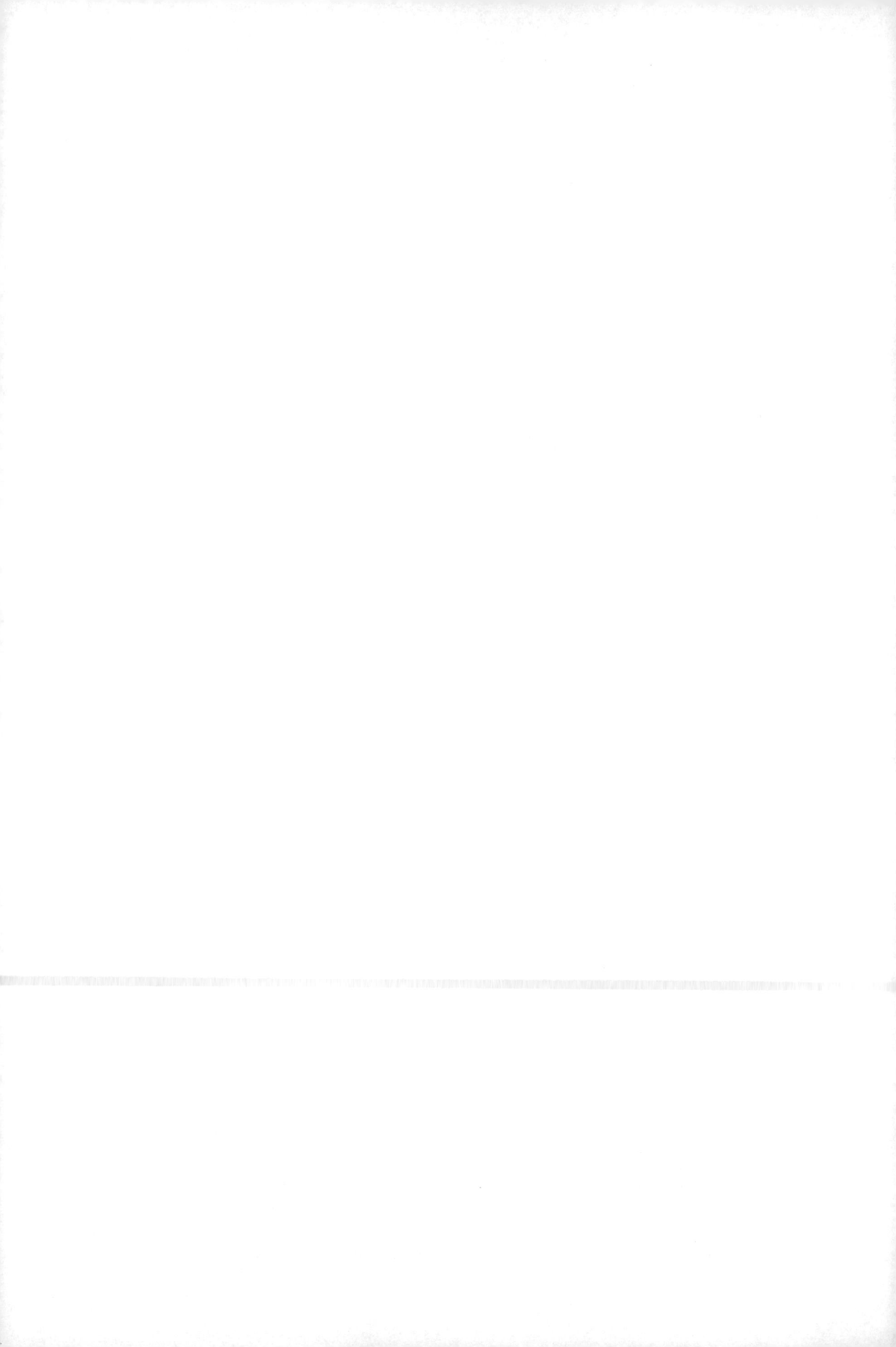

Index

A

Autoimmune hemolytic anemia (AIHA), 35–37

E

Enhanced recovery after surgery (ERAS)
- abdominal drainage tube removal, 55
- analgesia management, 55
- antithrombotic therapy, 53
- catheter removal timing, 56
- complications, 51
- discharge criteria, 56
- early postoperative activities, 55
- evidence-based medicine (EBM), 53
- incision selection, 54
- indications, 51
- intraoperative abdominal drainage tube placement, 54
- intraoperative hypothermia prevention, 54
- nasogastric tube indwelling, 53
- nutritional support therapy, 52
- perioperative period, 51
- postoperative nausea and vomiting prevention, 54
- postoperative nutritional support, 54
- preoperative education, 52
- preoperative fasting and water deprivation, 53
- preoperative nutrition screening, 52
- prophylactic use of antibiotics, 53
- stress-related mucosal disease (SRMD), 56

European Association for Endoscopic Surgery (EAES), 3

G

Gastroenterol perforation, 67

H

Hand-assisted laparoscopic splenectomy (HALS), 7, 9, 10
- advantages, 89, 90
- contraindications, 86
- disadvantages, 90
- hand port, 85
- imaging examination, 86
- indications, 86
- intraoperative circumstances and handling skills, 88
- patient assessment and preparation, 86
- physical examination, 86
- postoperative complications, 89
- postoperative management, 88
- surgical procedures, 86–88

Hemangioma of spleen, 44, 45

I

Immune thrombocytopenic purpura (ITP), 37–39

J

Japan Society for Endoscopic Surgery (JSES), 3

L

Laparoscopic partial splenectomy (LPS), 11–13
- contraindications, 94
- disadvantages, 101
- indications, 94, 99, 100
- intraoperative bleeding control, 100, 101
- intraoperative circumstances and handling skills, 97, 98
- minimally invasive surgery, 101
- post-operative complications, 98, 99
- post-operative management, 98
- pre-operative assessment, 102
- preoperative assessment and preparation, 94, 95
- splenic artery occlusion, 101
- surgical procedures, 95–97
- theoretical basis, 99

Laparoscopic splenectomy (LS)
- articles in PubMed, 1
- in children, 13, 15
- common benign blood disorders, 2
- contradictions, 59, 60
- contraindications, 6
- HALS, 7, 9, 10
- handling skills
  - autotransfusion, 64
  - Endo-GIA, 65
  - for severe abdominal adhesions, 64
  - for splenic pedicle, 64
  - for splenomegaly, 65

B. Peng (ed.), *Laparoscopic Surgery of the Spleen*, https://doi.org/10.1007/978-981-16-1216-9

Laparoscopic splenectomy (LS) *(cont.)*
  hematological disorders, 2
  indications, 1–6, 59
  liver cirrhosis and portal hypertension, 2–5
  long-term effects, 17
  LPS, 11–14
  occupying lesions, 3
  and open splenectomy (OS), 6–9
  postoperative complications, 7, 66–69
  postoperative management, 65, 66
  preoperative assessment and preparation, 60
  PVT, 15–17
  robot-assisted surgery, 17
  robotic splenectomy (RS), 11
  safety and effectiveness, 69
  SILS, 10, 11
  specimen removal specifications, 69, 70
  spleen injury, 3
  standard procedure, 17
  surgical position and surgeon position, 60–63
  surgical techniques, 63, 64
Laparoscopic splenectomy combined selective peripheral cardiac devascularization (LSSPD)
  adjacent organ injury, 108
  advantages, 110
  bleeding, 108
  blood autotransfusion, 108
  contraindications, 104
  disadvantages, 111
  hemostasis of surgical wound, 108
  indications, 103–104
  pericardial devascularization, 107
  postoperative management, 109
  preoperative assessment and preparation, 104–107
  prevention & treatment of complications, 109, 110
  selective pericardial devascularization, 110
LigaSure, 64
Lymphoma, 39, 40

O
Overwhelming post-splenectomy infection (OPSI), 67, 93

P
Pancreatic fistula, 101
Partial splenic embolization (PSE), 93
Portal hypertension (PH), 40–42
Portal venous thrombosis (PVT), 15–17

R
Radical antegrade modular pancreatosplenectomy (RAMPS)
  contraindications, 114, 115
  disadvantages, 123
  indications, 114
  inferior RAMPS, 113
  intraoperative circumstances and handling skills, 119, 120
  posterior RAMPS, 113
  postoperative management, 120–122
  preoperative assessment, 122
  preoperative assessment and preparation, 115
  R0 resection rate, 113, 114, 122, 123
  safety, 122
  surgical procedures, 115
    anatomical position and resection plane, 118
    drainage tube placement, 117–119
    exploration, 116
    inferior mesenteric vein treatment, 119
    local lymph node dissection, 116
    pancreas disconnection, 116, 117
    pancreas upper and lower edges dissection, 116
    renal veins and blood vessels protection, 119
    resection and cleaning of retroperitoneal tissue, 117
    spleen dissociation, 117, 118
    spleen movement, 116
    surgical position and trocar placement, 115, 116
    Treitz ligament approach, 116
    venous disconnection, 116
Robotic splenectomy (RS), 11

S
Single incision laparoscopic splenectomy (SILS)
  adjacent organ injury, 79
  advantages, 81
  contradictions, 74
  disadvantages, 81
  indications, 73
  intraoperative hemorrhage, 78, 79
  postoperative care, 79, 80
  postoperative complications, 80, 81
  preoperative assessment and preparation, 74
  surgical procedures, 74–78
Single-incision laparoscopic splenectomy (SILS), 10, 11
Spleen
  anterior spleen plica, 26
  congenital dysplasia
    accessory spleen, 21, 22
    asplenia and polysplenia, 22
    SGF, 23
    wandering spleen/ectopic spleen, 22, 23
  CT anatomy, 32
  division of, 29, 30
  double circulation pathway, 29
  embryology, 21
  gastrosplenic ligament, 24
  innervation, 30
  lienorenal ligament, 24, 25
  lobes and segments, 26
  lymphatic circulation, 30
  pancreaticocolic ligament, 26
  phrenicocolic ligament, 26
  physiology, 30, 31
  sectional anatomy, 26

- shape, position, and adjacency, 23, 24
- splenic artery, 27–29
- splenic notch, 26
- splenic vein, 29
- splenocolic ligament, 25
- splenophrenic ligament, 25
- ultrasonography anatomy, 31, 32

Splenic cyst, 43, 44
Splenic fever, 67
Splenic metastasis, 45
Splenic space-occupying lesions, 43
Splenic vein and portal vein thrombosis, 68
Splenogonadal fusion (SGF), 23

T

Traumatic splenic rupture, 46–48

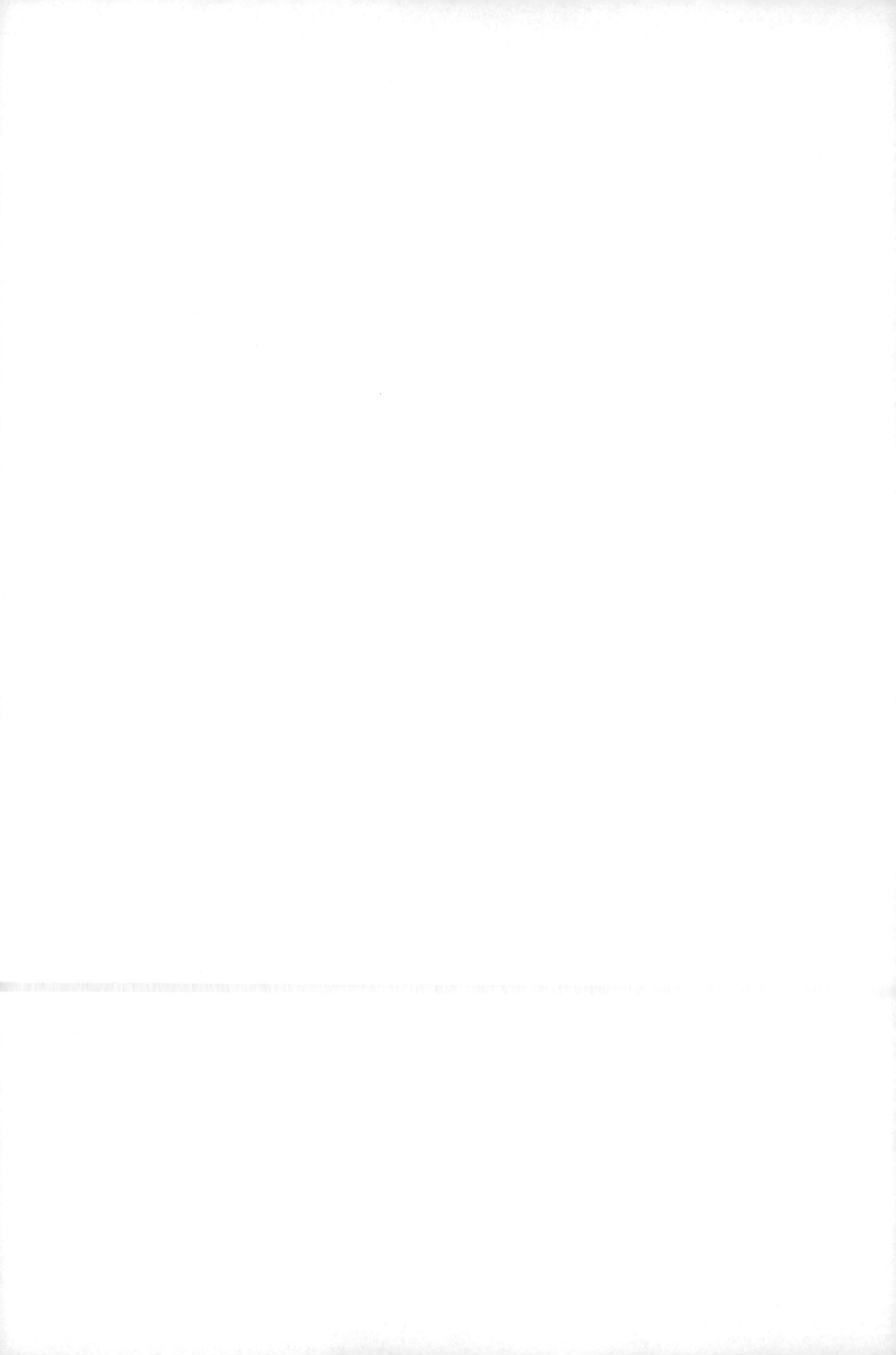

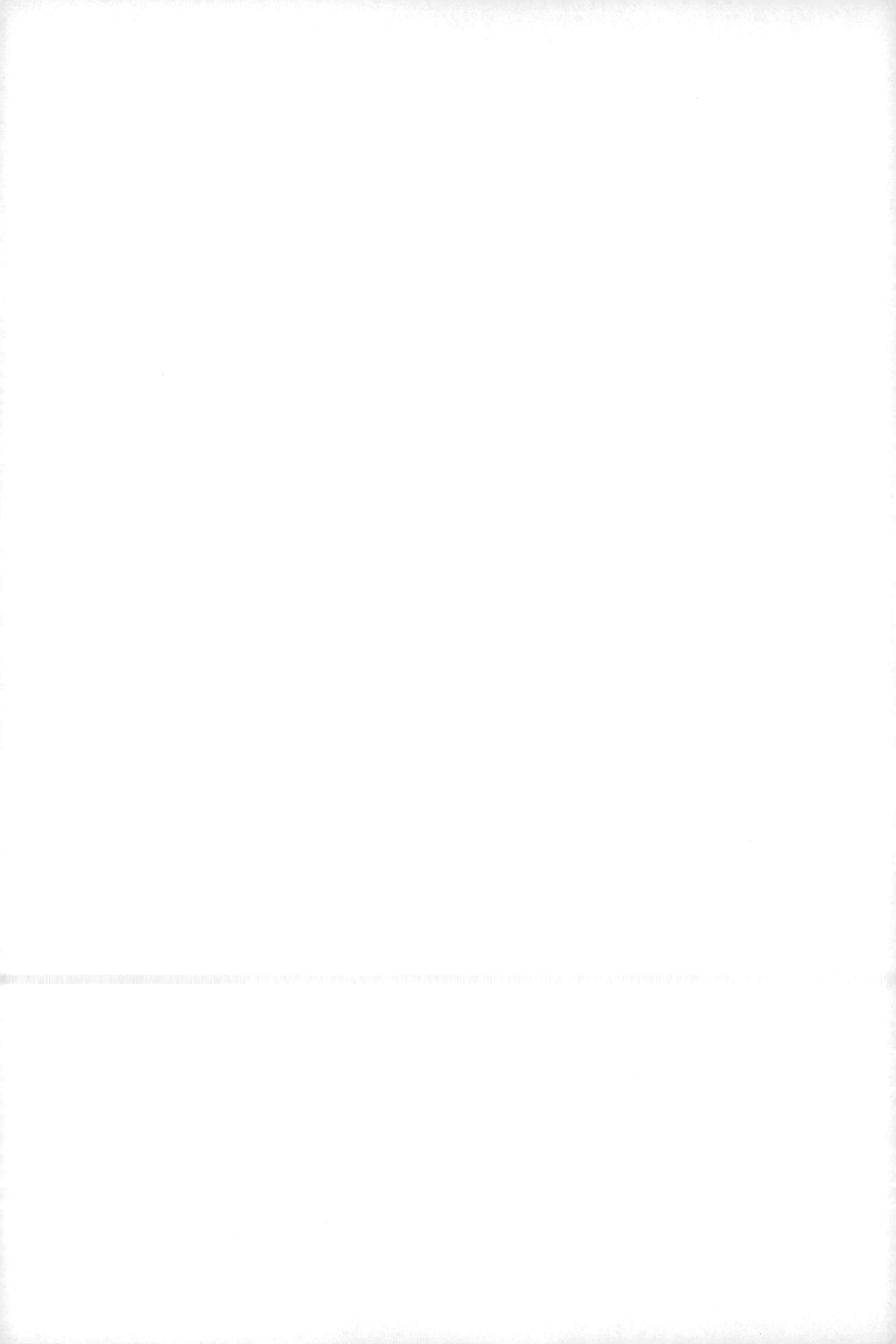

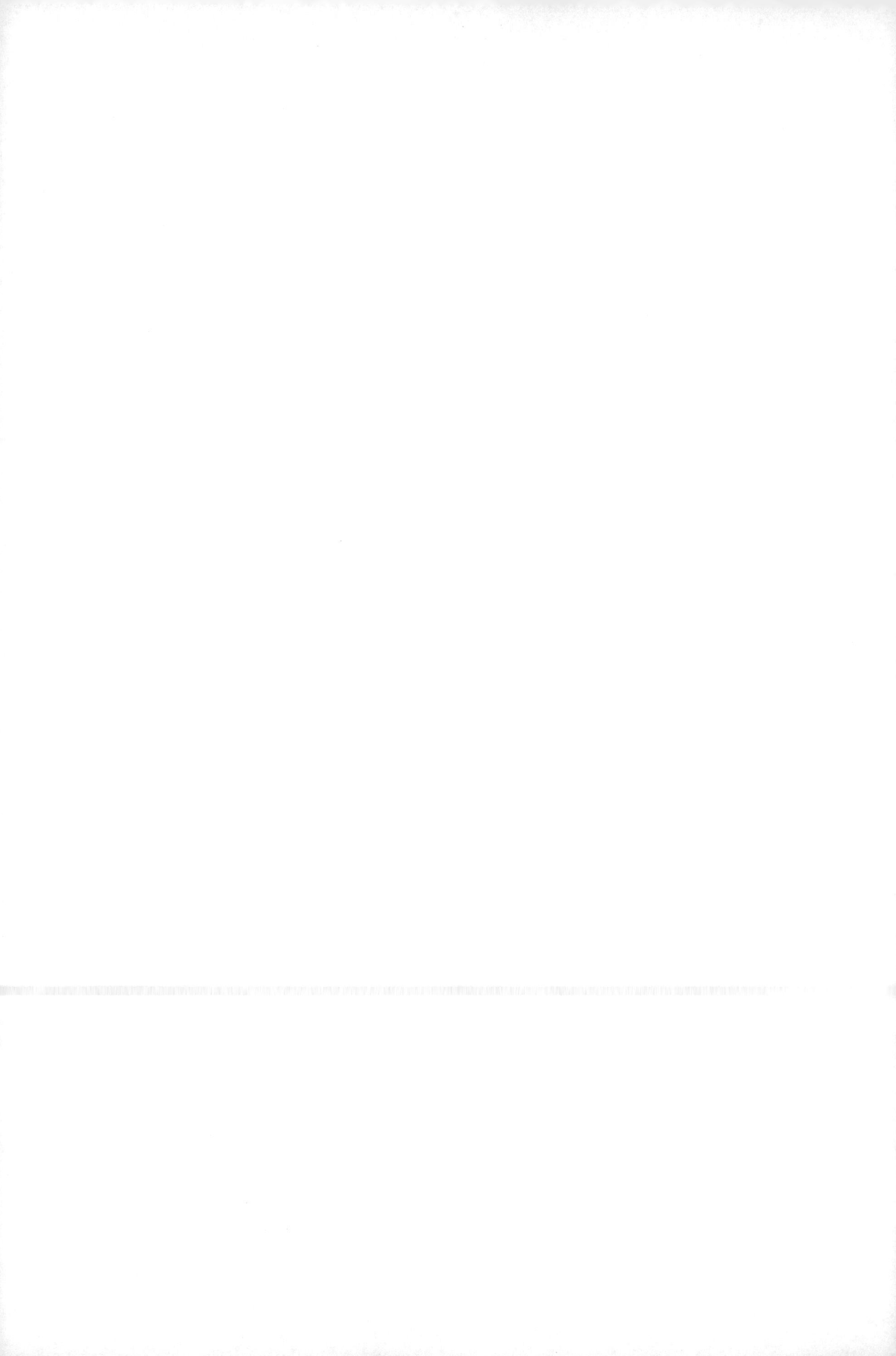

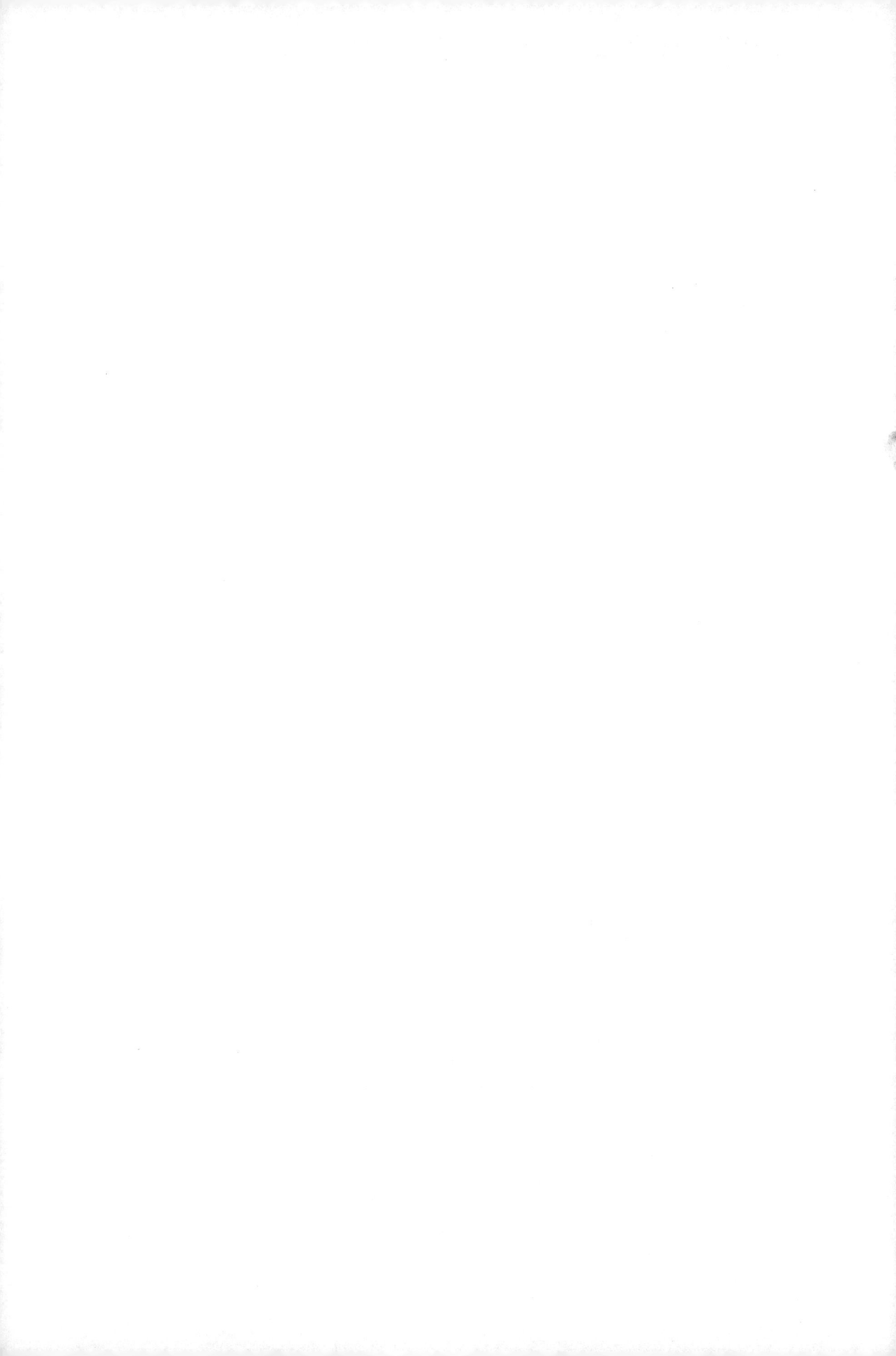

GPSR Compliance

The European Union's (EU) General Product Safety Regulation (GPSR) is a set of rules that requires consumer products to be safe and our obligations to ensure this.

If you have any concerns about our products, you can contact us on ProductSafety@springernature.com

In case Publisher is established outside the EU, the EU authorized representative is:

Springer Nature Customer Service Center GmbH
Europaplatz 3
69115 Heidelberg, Germany

Batch number: 10371063

Printed by Printforce, the Netherlands